A Medication Guide for Breastfeeding Moms

A Medication Guide
for Breastfeeding Moms

Thomas W. Hale, Ph.D.

Ghia McAfee, Ph.D.

Pharmasoft Publishing

A Medication Guide for Breastfeeding Moms

© Copyright 2005

Pharmasoft Publishing, L.P.

1712 N. Forest St.
Amarillo, TX   79106-7017
806-376-9900
800-378-1317

Disclaimer

The information contained in this publication is intended to supplement the knowledge of mothers regarding drug use during lactation. This information is advisory only and is not intended to replace sound clinical judgment or individualized patient care. The authors disclaim all warranties, whether expressed or implied, including any warranty as to the quality, accuracy, safety, or suitability of this information for any particular purpose.

ISBN 0-9729583-6-3

Library of Congress Control Number: 2005903793

Table of Contents

Preface

Worldwide, the interest in breastfeeding is growing enormously. More and more mothers across the world are now turning to breastmilk as the primary source of food for their babies. And the reason is simple: all the new research clearly shows that breastmilk is the finest nutrition a mother can give her newborn infant. Breastfeeding not only provides warmth and closeness, but also strengthens the mother-infant bond. But perhaps just as important, breastmilk provides an immune system for the baby's stomach and gut, which prevents the entry of harmful bacteria and disease. All the studies show the same thing, breastmilk saves the lives of babies time and again. However, not only the baby but also the mother benefit from breastfeeding. Figure 1 illustrates many of the benefits to infants and their mothers.

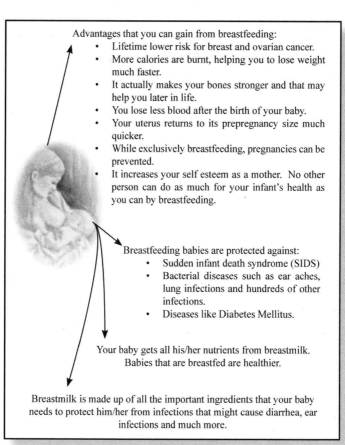

Advantages that you can gain from breastfeeding:
- Lifetime lower risk for breast and ovarian cancer.
- More calories are burnt, helping you to lose weight much faster.
- It actually makes your bones stronger and that may help you later in life.
- You lose less blood after the birth of your baby.
- Your uterus returns to its prepregnancy size much quicker.
- While exclusively breastfeeding, pregnancies can be prevented.
- It increases your self esteem as a mother. No other person can do as much for your infant's health as you can by breastfeeding.

Breastfeeding babies are protected against:
- Sudden infant death syndrome (SIDS)
- Bacterial diseases such as ear aches, lung infections and hundreds of other infections.
- Diseases like Diabetes Mellitus.

Your baby gets all his/her nutrients from breastmilk. Babies that are breastfed are healthier.

Breastmilk is made up of all the important ingredients that your baby needs to protect him/her from infections that might cause diarrhea, ear infections and much more.

Figure 1: Various advantages a mother and infant can gain from breastfeeding.

1

Whether you are pregnant or breastfeeding, you may be wondering whether you can safely take drugs. You are quite smart to think about this, since some drugs can harm babies in the womb and/or harm breastfeeding babies.

Sadly, one of the main reasons moms give for weaning is the use of drugs. Some doctors advise their patients to stop breastfeeding based only on the package insert that comes with the drug without checking to see if there are any reports in the medical journals on the effect of the drug on the fetus or breastfeeding infant. The drug company's information almost always cautions against use in breastfeeding to protect the company from law suits, not because of harmful effects to the infant. The fact is many drugs can be taken while breastfeeding without risk to the infant. What you need to know is which ones are going to harm your baby. Then, you can avoid these drugs.

Prescription drugs are not the only drugs that can cause problems. Over-the-counter drugs, herbs, and street drugs may contain substances that can harm a fetus or a breastfeeding baby. Check the entry in this book before you take any kind of drug! **The purpose of this book** is to provide information to you about the safety or possible harm of the drugs you might take.

In order to understand the content of this book, please read the following:

How do drugs reach the breastmilk?

When a mother takes a drug by mouth, it is absorbed into the body's bloodstream. Once the drug reaches the bloodstream, it is taken to the breast where small amounts may pass into milk. Figure 2 shows a single alveolus which makes milk and the artery that delivers drugs to the breast. A good rule is that the higher the amount of the drug in the mother's bloodstream, the more likely it is that more of the drug will enter the breastmilk. Also, the lower the amount in the mother's bloodstream, the less likely the drug will enter her milk.

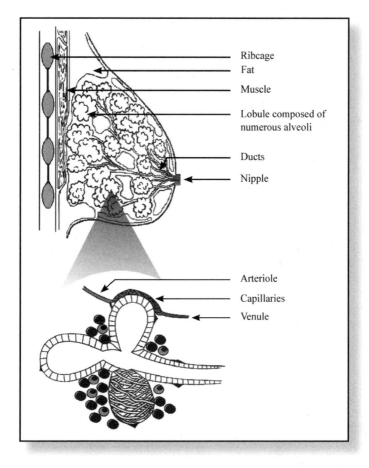

Figure 2: Drawing of the breast, indicating the alveolus, which makes milk, and its' blood supply.

What types of drugs are more likely to enter breastmilk?

Almost all drugs enter breastmilk to a limited degree, but the amount is most often low. With a few exceptions, the amount of drug the infant receives from breastfeeding is far less than the amount of the drug needed to produce a harmful effect.

Most drugs that transfer readily into breastmilk are:

- Highly fat soluble (meaning they dissolve in fats as opposed to water)
- Small molecules
- Able to pass into the brain easily
- Drugs that reach high levels in the mother's blood

Will the amount of drug that a breastfeeding infant receives cause an effect in the infant?

We believe that drugs in the mother's system pass into breastmilk more easily during the first three days after birth. However, the total amount of the drug the breastfeeding infant takes in is still thought to be low since the amount of the mother's first milk (colostrum) is small. By the end of the first week, the breast cells reduce the passage of most drugs into the breastmilk.

If the drug passes into the baby, will the baby absorb it?

Just because the drug passes into the baby does not mean that the drug will have an effect on the breastfeeding baby. Some drugs may be broken down in the baby's stomach acid before they can be absorbed, or they may be poorly absorbed into the baby's bloodstream. If the drug is absorbed by the infant's body, it may be broken down by the baby's liver and not cause an effect.

Of course, there are exceptions to this rule. Some drugs that enter the baby's stomach may cause diarrhea, constipation or even inflammation of the intestine, but this is rare.

Terms and abbreviations

You will see the following terms or abbreviations in the text:

<u>Drug name:</u>
> Each drug entry begins with the generic or chemical name of the drug.

<u>Trade names:</u>
> The USA, Canadian, Australian and United Kingdom trade names for the drug are provided.

<u>AAP recommendation:</u>
> The American Academy of Pediatrics provided recommendations in their document, *The transfer of drugs and other chemicals into human milk (Pediatrics. 2001 Sep;108(3):776-89.).*
> They have classified most drugs under one of the following:
> - Drugs that may harm the breastfeeding infant on a cellular level.
> - Drugs of abuse that have been reported to harm breastfeeding infants. These drugs are contraindicated

by the American Academy of Pediatrics in breastfeeding mothers.

- Radioactive compounds that require the mother to stop breastfeeding for a short period of time.
- Drug whose effect on nursing infants is unknown but may be of concern.
- Drug associated with significant side effects and should be taken with caution.
- Maternal medication usually compatible with breastfeeding.
- When drugs have not yet been reviewed by the AAP, "Not reviewed" will be noted. Most new drugs have not yet been reviewed.

Paragraph:

This section lists what is currently known about the drug and its ability to enter breastmilk.

Relative infant dose:

The percent of the mother's dose that an infant might receive from drinking his/her mother's milk. Generally, if it is less than 10%, it's probably safe to use.

Time to clear:

The time it will take for the mother's body to rid itself of the drug. After this time, little or no drug is left in the mother's body or in her milk. If you wait this long after taking a drug to breastfeed, little or no drug will enter your milk.

Lactation risk category:

We have defined five categories to show the relative risk of drugs in breastfeeding mothers and their infants. The categories defined below are a useful tool to show the possible risks associated with using the drug during breastfeeding. These risks may vary from one mother/infant to another, so close consultation with a doctor is advised.

 L1 (Safest):
Drug which has been taken by a large number of breastfeeding mothers without any observed increase in harmful effects to the infant. Controlled studies in breastfeeding women fail to show a risk to the infant, and it is unlikely to harm the breastfeeding infant. Or, the drug is not orally absorbed by the infant.

L2 (Safer):
Drug which has been studied in a limited number of breastfeeding women without an increase in harmful effects in the infant. And/or the chance of a harmful effect following the use of this drug is unlikely.

L3 (Moderately safe):
There are no controlled studies in breastfeeding women; however, there may be a risk of harmful effects in a breastfed infant. Or, controlled studies have shown only a few effects in breastfeeding infants, but they are only slight. These drugs should only be taken if the benefit to the mother justifies the risk to the infant.

L4 (May be harmful):
There is a risk to the breastfed infant or to breastmilk production. In some cases, the mother may have to take the drug despite the risk to the infant (e.g. if the drug is needed in a life-threatening situation or for a serious disease for which safer drugs cannot be used or are not effective).

L5 (Not to be used):
Studies in breastfeeding mothers have shown that the drug is harmful to the infant based on reports in humans. Or, it is a drug that has a high risk of causing major damage to an infant. The risk of using the drug in a breastfeeding woman clearly outweighs any possible benefit from breastfeeding. The drug should not be used by breastfeeding women.

Pregnancy risk category:

The Food and Drug Administration (FDA) has defined five categories to show the risk of drugs causing birth defects. Unfortunately, these categories do not state when during the pregnancy the drug is used. Some drugs are more harmful during certain trimesters of pregnancy. The categories defined below are a useful tool to show the possible risks linked with using the drug during pregnancy. The risk category for some of the newer drugs is not yet reported. In this case, the category will not be listed.

Although the FDA defined the categories, the drug company assigned the category to the drug. Note: the pregnancy risk category does not apply to breastfeeding.

Category A:
Controlled studies in women fail to show a risk to the fetus in the first trimester. No risk has been shown in later trimesters. There is little chance of harm to the fetus.

Category B:
Animal studies have not shown a risk to the fetus. There are no controlled studies in pregnant women or animals that have shown a harmful effect (other than a decrease in fertility) that was not confirmed in controlled studies in women in the first trimester. And, there is no proof of a risk in later trimesters.

Category C:
Either studies in animals have revealed harmful effects to the fetus and there are no controlled studies in women, or there are no studies in women and animals. These drugs should only be given if the benefit to the mother justifies the risk to the fetus

Category D:
There is positive proof of risk to the human fetus, but the benefits from use in pregnant women may be acceptable despite the risk (e.g. if the drug is needed in a life-threatening situation or for a serious disease and safer drugs cannot be used or are not effective).

Category X:
Studies in animals or humans have shown abnormalities in the fetus or there is evidence of a risk to the fetus based on human experience, or both. And, the risk of using the drug in pregnant women clearly outweighs any possible benefit. Women who are pregnant or who may become pregnant should not use this drug.

Adult dose:
The dose noted here is the usual adult oral dose provided in the package insert. While these are highly variable, the dose for the most common use of the medication was chosen.

Alternatives:
The listed drugs may be better choices for the mother to take. These drugs often act the same way, but we probably have good research studies showing they are safer or at least as good.
WARNING: The listed alternatives are only suggestions and may not be at all suitable for a specific condition. Only the doctor can make such a judgment.

Things to remember:

- Most drugs are probably quite safe in breastfeeding mothers. The risks of not breastfeeding and using infant formula are usually much higher for the infant.
- In spite of the fact that most drugs will not harm the breastfeeding infant, mothers should only take drugs when absolutely necessary. If you don't really need it, then please don't take it.
- As a general rule, if the relative infant dose is less than 10%, the drug is quite safe to use while breastfeeding. Note that the relative infant dose of most drugs is less than 1%.
- If possible, choose drugs with published reports as opposed to new drugs.
- Be slightly more concerned about using drugs in breastfeeding mothers with premature infants or newborns. The older the infant, the less the concern.
- Consult your doctor if you are receiving drugs in the hospital that are radioactive such as for a thyroid scan, etc. You may need to pump and discard your milk until the radioactive compounds are out of your system. Then you can continue breastfeeding.
- Finally, always remember to watch your infant for any changes in behavior or bowel habits once you start taking a drug. We don't always know how a specific infant may respond to a particular drug. Call your doctor if you notice changes that could be related to the drug you are taking.
- Please remember that human milk is the most perfect food you can give your infant. It also protects your infant from numerous diseases and is the best immunization you can give your infant. Don't give it up just because someone advises you to stop. It's simply too important to your infant's health. Always ask questions, resist advice to stop, and seek other experts input when necessary.

Thomas W. Hale Ph.D.
Ghia McAfee Ph.D.

Alphabetical Listing Of Medications

5-HYDROXYTRYPTOPHAN

Trade names: Powersleep, Oxitriptan

AAP recommendation: Not reviewed

5-Hydroxytryptophan (5-HTP) is an amino acid, a building block of protein. There is no information available on the transfer of 5-HTP into breastmilk. 5-HTP is rapidly absorbed by the mother and the infant. Approximately 70% of the dose is absorbed orally, the remaining 30% is converted to serotonin by intestinal cells. The infant's brain is very sensitive to serotonin. Because 5-HTP can increase serotonin levels in the brain, breastfeeding mothers should not use 5-HTP.

Relative infant dose:
Time to clear: Between 17 and 21.5 hours
Lactation risk category: L3
Pregnancy risk category:
Adult dose:
Alternatives:

ACARBOSE

Trade names: Precose, Prandase, Glucobay

AAP recommendation: Not reviewed

Acarbose is used for the treatment of Type II diabetes (noninsulin-dependent). Acarbose works by delaying the absorption of carbohydrates in the body, reducing the rapid rise in blood sugar (glucose) levels common after a meal. Very little acarbose taken by mouth is absorbed into the body. This reduces the amount of acarbose found in breastmilk and, therefore, taken in by the infant.

Relative infant dose:
Time to clear: Between 8 and 10 hours
Lactation risk category: L3
Pregnancy risk category: B
Adult dose: 50-100 milligrams three times daily
Alternatives:

ACEBUTOLOL

Trade names: Sectral

AAP recommendation: Maternal medication usually compatible with breastfeeding

Acebutolol is used to treat hypertension (high blood pressure) and is fairly well absorbed. Pregnant women with high blood pressure do well when taking acebutolol. Animal studies have shown that acebutolol does not appear to harm the fetus. Acebutolol and its major break down product (metabolite), diacetolol, do appear in breastmilk and newborn infants appear to be sensitive to acebutolol. Therefore, after birth other blood pressure lowering drugs should be used.

Relative infant dose: 3.6%
Time to clear: Between 12 and 20 hours
Lactation risk category: L3
Pregnancy risk category: B
Adult dose: 200-400 milligrams twice daily
Alternatives: Propranolol, Metoprolol

ACETAMINOPHEN

Trade names: Tempra, Tylenol, Paracetamol, Panadol, Dymadon, Calpol

AAP recommendation: Maternal medication usually compatible with breastfeeding

Acetaminophen is a well known pain killer. Acetaminophen is transferred into breastmilk at levels too small to be considered harmful. The amount of acetaminophen in breastmilk is much less than the amount that can be taken by infants for pain. Therefore, acetaminophen is more than likely safe for breastfeeding mothers.

Relative infant dose: 6.4%
Time to clear: Between 8 and 10 hours
Lactation risk category: L1
Pregnancy risk category: B
Adult dose: 325-650 milligrams every 4-6 hours as needed
Alternatives:

ACETAZOLAMIDE

Trade names: Dazamide, Diamox, Apo-Acetazolamide

AAP recommendation: Maternal medication usually compatible with breastfeeding

Acetazolamide is a drug that increases the flow of urine (a diuretic). It is thought that diuretics may decrease milk volume, but this is not known for sure. Acetazolamide is transferred into breastmilk, but it is unlikely to cause harmful effects in the infant.

Relative infant dose: 2.2%
Time to clear: Between 9.5 and 29 hours
Lactation risk category: L2
Pregnancy risk category: C
Adult dose: 500 milligrams twice daily
Alternatives:

ACYCLOVIR

Trade names: Zovirax, Aviraz, Apo-Acyclovir, Acyclo-V, Zyclir, Aciclover

AAP recommendation: Maternal medication usually compatible with breastfeeding

Acyclovir is used to treat viral infections, which include herpes simplex and varicella zoster (chicken pox). Herpes simplex virus type 1 (HSV-1) causes cold sores around the mouth area. Herpes simplex virus type 2 (HSV-2) causes blisters in the genital area. These infections can be treated with acyclovir cream or ointment applied on the infected area. Very little is absorbed when applied to the skin. While acyclovir is present in milk, the levels are not high enough to affect the infant. Acyclovir is commonly used in pediatric units in hospitals and produces few toxicities.

Relative infant dose: 1.5%
Time to clear: Between 9.5 and 12 hours
Lactation risk category: L2
Pregnancy risk category: C
Adult dose: 200-800 milligrams every 4-6 hours
Alternatives:

ADAPALENE

Trade names: Differin
AAP recommendation: Not reviewed

Adapalene is used to treat acne. Since this drug is applied to the skin as a cream, gel, or solution, very little is absorbed by the body. There are no reports on the transfer of adapalene into breastmilk. Since adapalene is applied to the skin of the mother and is largely unabsorbed, the mother's blood levels of adapalene are almost nil. Therefore, the levels of adapalene in breastmilk would likely be very low.

Relative infant dose:
Time to clear:
Lactation risk category: L3
Pregnancy risk category: C
Adult dose: Apply topically daily
Alternatives: Tretinoin

ALBUTEROL

Trade names: Proventil, Ventolin, Asmavent, Respax,
Respolin, Asmol, Salbulin, Salbuvent, Salamol
AAP recommendation: Not reviewed

Albuterol is used to relieve the symptoms patients have during asthma attacks. It can be taken orally (by mouth) in tablet form or, more commonly, inhaled through an inhaler. If albuterol is taken by mouth, it may be transferred into breastmilk and could cause tremors and agitation in the infant. If a breastfeeding mother uses an albuterol inhaler, small amounts (10%) of albuterol are absorbed into her bloodstream. This amount, if transferred into breastmilk, would be unlikely to produce an effect in the infant. Inhaled albuterol is commonly used for the treatment of pediatric asthma and is, therefore, safe to use in breastfeeding mothers and infants.

Relative infant dose:
Time to clear: Between 15 and 19 hours
Lactation risk category: L1
Pregnancy risk category: C
Adult dose: 2-4 milligrams three or four times daily
Alternatives:

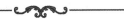

ALBUTEROL AND IPRATROPIUM BROMIDE

Trade names: DuoNeb

AAP recommendation: Not reviewed

Duo Neb is a product which contains both albuterol and ipratropium bromide. See the entry for each drug for more information.

Relative infant dose:
Time to clear:
Lactation risk category:
Pregnancy risk category:
Adult dose:
Alternatives:

ALENDRONATE SODIUM

Trade names: Fosamax

AAP recommendation: Not reviewed

Alendronate is used in men and women to treat and prevent osteoporosis. These drugs stay in bone for long periods stopping bone loss. Although there are no reports on the transfer of alendronate into breastmilk, it is unlikely to occur. Alendronate is poorly absorbed by the body of the breastfeeding infant because it is ingested with milk. Since we do not know if even small amounts of this drug are safe in a breastfed infant, use with caution.

Relative infant dose:
Time to clear: Between 12 and 15 hours
Lactation risk category: L3
Pregnancy risk category: C
Adult dose: 10 milligrams daily
Alternatives:

ALFENTANIL

Trade names: Alfenta, Rapifen

AAP recommendation: Not reviewed

Alfentanil is a strong pain killer used before, after and during surgery. Although it is transferred into breastmilk, the levels are likely to be too low to cause a lot of side effects in breastfeeding infants.

Relative infant dose: 4.7%
Time to clear: Between 4 and 10 hours
Lactation risk category: L2
Pregnancy risk category: C
Adult dose: 8-40 micrograms per kilogram total
Alternatives: Remifentanil

ALLERGY INJECTIONS

Trade names:

AAP recommendation: Not reviewed

Allergy injections consist of protein and carbohydrate substances from plants and animals. Allergy injections are unlikely to be transferred into breastmilk. There have been no reported ill effects in breastfeeding infants.

Relative infant dose:
Time to clear:
Lactation risk category: L1
Pregnancy risk category:
Adult dose:
Alternatives:

ALMOTRIPTAN

Trade names: Axert, Almogran

AAP recommendation: Not reviewed

Almotriptan is used to treat migraine headaches. There are no reports on the transfer of almotriptan into breastmilk. Sumatriptan, another drug commonly used to treat migraine attacks, has been well studied in breastfeeding women and may be a better drug to use.

Relative infant dose:
Time to clear: Between 12 and 20 hours
Lactation risk category: L3
Pregnancy risk category: C
Adult dose: 6.25-12.5 milligrams
Alternatives: Sumatriptan

ALOE VERA

Trade names: Aloe Vera, Cape, Zanzibar, Socotrine

AAP recommendation: Not reviewed

There are over 500 species of aloe. The plant yields two main products: Aloe latex made from the outer skin of the plant and Aloe gel made from the inner tissue of the leaf. Aloe latex, a bitter yellow product, is a very strong laxative and should not be taken by mouth by children or pregnant women. Aloe latex is used in burn therapy for minor burns and skin irritations, but studies do not show that it works better than good wound care. Aloe gel is most commonly used in cosmetics and health food products. The topical use of aloe gel is safe for breastfeeding mothers.

Relative infant dose:
Time to clear:
Lactation risk category: L3
Pregnancy risk category:
Adult dose:
Alternatives:

ALOSETRON

Trade names: Lotronex

AAP recommendation: Not reviewed

Alosetron is only used to treat severe diarrhea - predominant irritable bowel syndrome (IBS) in women with chronic symptoms who meet specific requirements. There are no reports on the transfer of alosetron into breastmilk. Alesteron does not stay in the body for a long time, but the by-products that form after alosteron is broken down remain for a longer time. The importance of these by-products is unknown. Less than 25% of alosetron is absorbed by the body if the drug is taken with food. Therefore, it is unlikely that levels of alosetron will be very high in breastmilk or that they will produce side effects in the infant.

Relative infant dose:
Time to clear: Between 6 and 7.5 hours
Lactation risk category: L3
Pregnancy risk category: B
Adult dose: 1 milligram twice daily
Alternatives:

ALPRAZOLAM

Trade names: Xanax, Novo-Alprazol, Kalma, Ralozam

AAP recommendation: Drug whose effect on nursing infants is unknown but may be of concern

Alprazolam is used to treat anxiety and panic disorders. Infants have been reported to suffer from minor withdrawal symptoms (irritability, crying, and sleep disturbances) after long term exposure through breastmilk. As a rule, this family of drugs is not ideal for breastfeeding mothers if used long-term. However, some shorter-acting sedatives in this family are safer during lactation if their use is short-term or used every now and then, in low doses, and after the first week of life.

Relative infant dose: 7.8%
Time to clear: Between 2 and 3 days
Lactation risk category: L3
Pregnancy risk category: D
Adult dose: 0.5-1 milligram three times daily
Alternatives: Lorazepam

AMIKACIN

Trade names: Amikin

AAP recommendation: Not reviewed

Amikacin is an antibiotic and is available as an injection. Only small amounts, if any, are transferred into breastmilk. Other antibiotics in the same class are poorly absorbed by the body, but they can produce changes in gastrointestinal flora in the infant leading to diarrhea. In a small study of patients who received amikacin, none to trace amounts were found in breastmilk.

Relative infant dose:
Time to clear: Between 9 and 11.5 hours
Lactation risk category: L2
Pregnancy risk category: C
Adult dose: 5-7.5 milligrams/kilogram/dose three times daily
Alternatives:

AMINOSALICYLIC ACID (PARA)

Trade names: Paser, PAS, Nemasol

AAP recommendation: Drug associated with significant side effects and should be taken with caution

Aminosalicylic acid (PARA) is used to treat tuberculosis and ulcerative colitis. PARA enters breastmilk, but the amount is too low to produce major problems in most infants. If you are taking PARA, observe the infant for diarrhea. There has been one report of slight diarrhea in one infant.

Relative infant dose: 0.3%
Time to clear: Between 4 and 5 hours
Lactation risk category: L3
Pregnancy risk category: C
Adult dose: 150 milligrams/kilogram/day two or three times daily
Alternatives:

AMITRIPTYLINE

Trade names: Elavil, Endep, Novo-Tryptin, Amitrol, Mutabon D, Tryptanol, Domical, Lentizol

AAP recommendation: Drug whose effect on nursing infants is unknown but may be of concern

Amitriptyline is used to treat a major depressive disorder and many chronic pain syndromes. Amitriptyline is broken down to form nortriptyline. Both amitriptyline and nortriptyline are transferred into breastmilk in small amounts. The amount the infant will absorb is unlikely to cause problems. Several studies have been done and their authors suggest the risk to the infant is very low.

Relative infant dose: 1.5%
Time to clear: Between 5 and 9.5 days
Lactation risk category: L2
Pregnancy risk category: D
Adult dose: 15-150 milligrams twice daily
Alternatives: Amoxapine, Imipramine

AMOXAPINE

Trade names: Asendin, Asendis

AAP recommendation: Drug whose effect on nursing infants is unknown but may be of concern

Amoxapine is used to treat major depressive disorders. Amoxapine and its break down products are transferred into breastmilk at low levels. Several studies of this drug do not suggest it produces major problems for a breastfed infant.

Relative infant dose: 0.5%
Time to clear: Between 32 and 40 hours
Lactation risk category: L2
Pregnancy risk category: C
Adult dose: 25 milligrams two or three times daily
Alternatives:

AMOXICILLIN

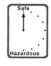

Trade names: Larotid, Amoxil, Apo-Amoxi, Novamoxin, Alphamox, Moxacin, Cilamox, Betamox

AAP recommendation: Maternal medication usually compatible with breastfeeding

Amoxicillin is an antibiotic used to treat otitis media (middle ear infection) and many other infections in children and adults. Amoxicillin is transferred into breastmilk (1.0% of the mother's dose), but no harmful effects have been reported in breastfeeding infants. Stool changes such as diarrhea are possible but unlikely. This medication is thought to be safe in most instances.

Relative infant dose: 1.0%
Time to clear: Between 7 and 8.5 hours
Lactation risk category: L1
Pregnancy risk category: B
Adult dose: 500-875 milligrams twice daily
Alternatives:

AMOXICILLIN AND CLAVULANATE

Trade names: Augmentin, Clavulin

AAP recommendation: Not reviewed

Giving clavulanate with amoxicillin ensures that amoxicillin is protected from certain bacterial enzymes that destroy it before it can act on the bacteria. There are no reports on the transfer of clavulanate into breastmilk, although, only small amounts should transfer. It may cause changes in gastrointestinal bacteria and may lead to fungal (candida) overgrowth. Amoxicillin is the most common antibiotic used in infants.

Relative infant dose: 1.0%
Time to clear: Between 7 and 8.5 hours
Lactation risk category: L1
Pregnancy risk category: B
Adult dose: 875 milligrams twice daily
Alternatives:

AMPHETAMINES, HALLUCINOGENIC

Trade names: Ecstasy, Adam, Eve, Harmony, Love

AAP recommendation: Contraindicated by the American Academy of Pediatrics in breastfeeding mothers

This class of drugs includes the following which are known by their "street names" as Adam, Ecstasy, XTC, Essence, Eve, Harmony, Love, Love Drug and Speed for Lovers. All of these drugs can produce extreme hallucinations and possess severe stimulant activity. Large amounts of these drugs may transfer into breastmilk. The infant could have hallucinations, extreme agitation, and seizures if exposed right after the drug is taken.

It is not known when it is safe to start breastfeeding again, but 24-48 hours should be long enough to reduce the risks to the infant. The length of time depends on the amount of the drug taken by the mother. Breastfeeding mothers should not use these drugs, but if she does, she should pump and discard her milk until these drugs are out of her system (24-48 hours).

Relative infant dose:
Time to clear: Between 32 and 40 hours
Lactation risk category: L5
Pregnancy risk category:
Adult dose:

Alternatives:

AMPICILLIN

Trade names: Polycillin, Omnipen, Novo-Ampicillin, NuAmpi, Penbriton, Ampicyn, Austrapen, Amfipen, Britcin, Vidopen

AAP recommendation: Not reviewed

Ampicillin is an antibiotic used to treat a wide range of infections. Only small amounts transfer into human milk. Ampicillin has not been detected in the blood (plasma) of any infant. Possible rash, sensitization, diarrhea or candida overgrowth can occur in the infant, although it is unlikely. Antibiotics commonly change the bacteria in the gastrointestinal tract leading to diarrhea in some infants. Ampicillin is one of the most commonly used antibiotics in pediatric nurseries. In newborns, ampicillin is cleared from the body in 3 to 4 hours.

Relative infant dose: 1.5%
Time to clear: Between 5 and 6.5 hours
Lactation risk category: L1
Pregnancy risk category: B
Adult dose: 250-500 milligrams four times daily
Alternatives: Amoxicillin

AMPICILLIN AND SULBACTAM

Trade names: Unasyn, Dicapen

AAP recommendation: Not reviewed

Giving sulbactam with ampicillin ensures that ampicillin is protected from enzymes that destroy it before it can act on the bacteria. There are no reports on the levels of sulbactam in breastmilk, but the amount is probably very low. Ampicillin may cause possible rash, sensitization, diarrhea or candidiasis in the infant, although it is unlikely.

Relative infant dose: 1.5%
Time to clear: Between 5 and 6.5 hours
Lactation risk category: L1
Pregnancy risk category: B
Adult dose: 1.5-3 grams four times daily

Alternatives:

ANTHRALIN

Trade names: Anthra-Derm, Drithocreme, Dritho-Scalp, Micanol, Anthranol, Anthrascalp, Dithranol, Alphodith

AAP recommendation: Not reviewed

Anthralin is used to treat psoriasis (reddish, silvery-scaled lesions which occur mainly on the elbows, knees, scalp and trunk). Anthralin comes in the form of a cream and is applied to the affected areas. Anthralin cream can stain the skin and permanently stain clothing and porcelain bathroom fixtures. Only small amounts of anthralin enter the body after it is applied to the skin. There are no reports on the transfer of anthralin into breastmilk.

Applying anthralin cream on the nipples of breastfeeding mothers is discouraged. When a breastfeeding mother starts intense treatment over a large area of the body (arm, trunk, leg), it might be wise to stop breastfeeding and pump and discard the milk for 24 hours; although, this may be overly conservative. Observe the infant for diarrhea. Anthralin has been used in children over 2 years of age for the treatment of psoriasis.

Relative infant dose:
Time to clear:
Lactation risk category: L3
Pregnancy risk category: C
Adult dose: Apply topically twice daily
Alternatives:

ARGININE

Common names: L-Arginine, Arginine

AAP recommendation: Not reviewed

L-Arginine is an amino acid and is found in most foods. There are no reports on the transfer of l-arginine in breastmilk. As this product is not very useful in most patients, high doses in breastfeeding mothers should be avoided.

Relative infant dose:
Time to clear: Between 8 and 10 hours
Lactation risk category: L3
Pregnancy risk category: B

Adult dose: 1-2 grams per day but highly variable. Doses as high as 30 grams per day have been used short-term.
Alternatives:

ARIPIPRAZOLE

Trade names: Abilify
AAP recommendation: Not reviewed

Aripiprazole is used to treat schizophrenia (a type of psychosis). At this time, other drugs such as risperidone and olanzapine are preferred due to published reports in breastfeeding mothers.

Relative infant dose:
Time to clear: Between 12.5 and 15.5 days
Lactation risk category: L3
Pregnancy risk category: C
Adult dose: 10-15 milligrams per day
Alternatives: Risperidone, Olanzapine

ASCORBIC ACID

Trade names: Ascorbica, Cecon, Cevi-Bid, Ce-Vi-Sol,
                            Vitamin C
AAP recommendation: Not reviewed

Ascorbic acid, also known as vitamin C, is found in breastmilk. Moderate Vitamin C intake in the mother does not alter (or increase) the controlled amount secreted into breastmilk; although, very high doses may increase milk levels. The recommended daily dose of ascorbic acid for breastfeeding mothers is 100 milligrams per day. Pregnant women should not take excess amounts of ascorbic acid because it causes the fetal liver to metabolize vitamin C faster, followed by a rebound scurvy after birth.

Ascorbic acid should not be given to breastfed infants unless the infant is treated for scurvy. Scurvy is the dietary lack of vitamin C. Symptoms of scurvy include swollen and bleeding gums, bleeding under the skin and deep tissues, anemia (below normal levels of red blood cells and/or hemoglobin), and sore, stiff joints.

Relative infant dose:
Time to clear:
Lactation risk category: L1

Pregnancy risk category: A during 1st and 2nd trimester
C during 3rd trimester
Adult dose: 45-60 milligrams daily
Alternatives:

ASPARTAME

Trade names: Nutrasweet

AAP recommendation: Not reviewed

Aspartame is an artificial sweetener. Once in the gut, it is quickly changed to phenylalanine and aspartic acid, two normal amino acids found in all foods. Aspartame is transferred into breastmilk, but the level is likely to be too low to produce problems in normal infants. It should not be used in breastfeeding mothers with infants with proven phenylketonuria (PKU).

Relative infant dose:
Time to clear:
Lactation risk category: L1
L5 if used in infants with PKU
Pregnancy risk category: B
Adult dose:
Alternatives:

ASPIRIN

Trade names: Anacin, Aspergum, Empirin, Genprin,
Ecotrin, Arthritis Foundataion Pain Reliever, Novasen,
Entrophen, Disprin, Aspro, Cartia

AAP recommendation: Drug associated with significant side effects and
should be taken with caution

Aspirin is a well known pain killer. Only a small amount is transferred into breastmilk and few harmful effects have been reported. Very high doses taken by the mother may produce slight bleeding in the infant. Since there is a link between aspirin and Reye's Syndrome in the infant, aspirin is a poor choice for breastfeeding mothers. However, in patients with rheumatic fever, it is still the drug of choice, and the risks versus the benefits should be assessed in this case. Ibuprofen and acetaminophen are better choices for pain relief in the breastfeeding mother.

Relative infant dose: 0.04%

Time to clear: Between 10 and 35 hours
Lactation risk category: L3
Pregnancy risk category: C during 1st and 2nd trimester
D during 3rd trimester
Adult dose: 325-900 milligrams four times daily
Alternatives: Ibuprofen, Acetaminophen

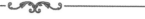

ATENOLOL

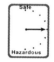

Trade names: Tenoretic, Tenormin, Anselol, Noten, Tenlol, Tensig, Antipress

AAP recommendation: Drug associated with significant side effects and should be taken with caution

Atenolol is used to treat hypertension (high blood pressure) or chronic stable angina pectoris (heart cramps) in patients with Type 1 diabetes mellitus or chronic obstructive pulmonary disease (COPD). The reports on the transfer of atenolol in breastmilk conflict. One study reported harmful side effects in breastfeeding infants including slow heart rate, cyanosis (low levels of oxygen in the blood), low body temperature, and low blood pressure. Although atenolol is approved by the American Academy of Pediatrics (AAP), use with some caution.

Relative infant dose: 6.6%
Time to clear: Between 24.5 and 30.5 hours
Lactation risk category: L3
Pregnancy risk category: C
Adult dose: 50-100 milligrams daily
Alternatives: Propranolol, Metoprolol

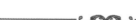

ATOMOXETINE

Trade names: Strattera

AAP recommendation: Not reviewed

Atomoxetine is used to treat attention-deficit hyperactivity disorder (ADHD). There are no reports on the transfer of atomoxetine into breastmilk. When taking the chemical properties of atomoxetine into account, there could be a risk for breastfeeding infants. Breastfeeding mothers should use with caution.

Relative infant dose:

Time to clear: Between 21 and 26 hours
Lactation risk category: L4
Pregnancy risk category: C
Adult dose: 0.5-1.2 milligrams per kilogram per day
Alternatives:

ATORVASTATIN CALCIUM

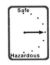

Trade names: Lipitor

AAP recommendation: Not reviewed

Atorvastatin is used to treat hypercholesterolemia (high cholesterol). There are no reports on the transfer of atorvastatin into breastmilk. Since cholesterol and other compounds are needed for fetal and newborn development, breastfeeding mothers should not use cholesterol-lowering drugs for any reason.

Relative infant dose:
Time to clear: Between 2.5 and 3 days
Lactation risk category: L3
Pregnancy risk category: X
Adult dose: 10-80 milligrams daily
Alternatives:

ATROPINE

Trade names: Belladonna, Atropine, Atropisol, Atropt,
Isopto-Atropine, Eyesule

AAP recommendation: Maternal medication usually compatible with
breastfeeding

Atropine has a wide range of uses, including the treatment of peptic ulcer disease, irritable bowel syndrome, and as medication before surgery. Only small amounts are believed to be transferred into breastmilk. Use with caution or avoid if infant is younger than one month because they can be very sensitive to it.

Relative infant dose:
Time to clear: Between 17 and 21.5 hours
Lactation risk category: L3
Pregnancy risk category: C
Adult dose: 0.6 milligrams every 6 hours

Alternatives:

AZAPROPAZONE

Trade names: Rheumox
AAP recommendation: Maternal medication usually compatible with breastfeeding

Azapropazone is used as pain relief in cases where inflammation is involved, such as gout, arthritis, and ankylosing spondylitis (a certain type of arthritis). Azapropazone levels in milk are low. Only about 2% of the mother's dose reaches the infant. No side effects have been reported in breastfeeding infants.

Relative infant dose:	2.1%
Time to clear:	Between 2 and 3 days
Lactation risk category:	L2
Pregnancy risk category:	
Adult dose:	600 milligrams twice daily
Alternatives:	Celecoxib

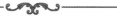

AZATHIOPRINE

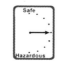

Trade names: Imuran, Thioprine
AAP recommendation: Not reviewed

Azathioprine is used for kidney transplants to prevent the body from rejecting the new kidney and in the treatment of severe rheumatoid arthritis which does not respond to other drugs. In the body, azathioprine is broken down to form 6-mercaptopurine which is transferred into breastmilk. In one study, the authors concluded that the level of 6-mercaptopurine in breastmilk is likely to be too low to produce any side effects in a breastfed infant.

One infant who was breastfed during therapy, displayed no immuno-suppressive effects. In another study, two infants were breastfed by mothers receiving 75-100 milligrams per day azathioprine. Both infants had normal blood counts, no increase in infections, and above-average growth rate. But, caution is suggested when using this potent drug.

Relative infant dose:	0.3%
Time to clear:	Between 2.5 and 3 hours
Lactation risk category:	L3
Pregnancy risk category:	D

Adult dose: 1-2.5 milligrams per kilogram per day
Alternatives:

AZELAIC ACID

Trade names: Azelex, Finevin, Skinoren
AAP recommendation: Not reviewed

Azelaic acid is found in whole grains and animal products. Azelaic acid, when applied as a cream, is used in the treatment of acne. When it is applied as a gel, it is used to treat inflammatory lesions caused by mild to moderate rosacea in adults. Small amounts of azelaic acid are normally present in human milk. However, less than 4% azelaic acid is absorbed by the body after it is applied to the skin. Due to the poor entry into plasma and rapid half-life (45 min.), it is not likely to enter breastmilk or produce ill effects in a breastfed infant.

Relative infant dose:
Time to clear: Between 3 and 4 hours
Lactation risk category: L3
Pregnancy risk category: B
Adult dose: Apply topically twice daily
Alternatives:

AZELASTINE

Trade names: Astelin, Optivar, Azep, Rhinolast, Optilast
AAP recommendation: Not reviewed

Azelastine comes as a nasal spray, tablet, or eye drops. The eye drops are used to treat rhinitis (inflammation of the nasal mucous membrane), nonallergic rhinitis, and conjunctivitis (itchy eyes). There are no reports on the transfer of azelastine into breastmilk. However, the amount of azelastine received in a nasal spray or eye drops is so low that it is very unlikely to produce levels in breastmilk high enough to cause problems in the infant.

If given orally, there may be slightly higher levels in the body, but azelastine has no serious side effects. However, this is a very bitter product and even tiny amounts in milk could alter the taste of milk leading the infant to reject the breast.

Relative infant dose:
Time to clear: Between 3.5 and 4.5 days

Lactation risk category: L3
Pregnancy risk category: C
Adult dose: Variable: 1-2 sprays (137 micrograms per spray) per nostril twice daily
Alternatives: Loratadine, Cetirizine

AZITHROMYCIN

Trade names: Zithromax
AAP recommendation: Not reviewed

Azithromycin is used to treat mild to moderate upper and lower respiratory tract infections as well as some skin infections. Azithromycin is transferred into breastmilk. However, the amount of azithromycin the infant receives from breastfeeding is very small - approximately 0.4 milligrams per kilogram per day.

Relative infant dose: < 2.9%
Time to clear: Between 8 and 14 days
Lactation risk category: L2
Pregnancy risk category: B
Adult dose: 250-500 milligrams daily
Alternatives:

BARIUM

Trade names: Barium, Medebar, Medescan, Baritop
AAP recommendation: Not reviewed

Barium is used as a contrast agent in X-rays or other forms of penetrating radiation. The amount of barium absorbed by the breastfeeding mother's body is limited. No harmful effects have been reported in breastfeeding infants.

Relative infant dose:
Time to clear:
Lactation risk category: L1
Pregnancy risk category:
Adult dose:
Alternatives:

BECLOMETHASONE

Trade names: Vanceril, Beclovent, Beconase, Becloforte, Aldecin, Becotide, Propadem

AAP recommendation: Not reviewed

Beclomethasone is used to treat rhinitis (inflammation of the nasal mucous membrane), nasal polyposis (growths inside of the nose), and asthma. Beclomethasone is available as an inhaler or in intranasal sprays. Because only small amounts of beclomethasone are absorbed, the transfer of beclomethasone into breastmilk is small. It is unlikely that an infant will receive harmful amounts of beclomethasone from breastfeeding.

Relative infant dose:
Time to clear: Between 2.5 and 3 days
Lactation risk category: L2
Pregnancy risk category: C
Adult dose: 504-840 micrograms daily
Alternatives:

BENAZEPRIL HCL

Trade names: Lotensin, Lotrel

AAP recommendation: Not reviewed

Benazepril is used to treat high blood pressure, congestive heart failure, and kidney disease. Benazepril is poorly absorbed by the body (37%), and therefore, only small amounts transfer into breastmilk. The infant receives a very small amount of benazepril through breastfeeding (less than 0.1% of the maternal dose). Benazepril belongs to the ACE inhibitor family. Lotrel is a combination product containing benazepril and amlodipine, a calcium channel blocker.

Relative infant dose:
Time to clear: Between 1.5 and 2.5 days
Lactation risk category: L3
Pregnancy risk category: D
Adult dose: 20-40 milligrams daily
Alternatives: Enalapril, Captopril

BEPRIDIL HCL

Trade names: Vascor, Bepadin

AAP recommendation: Not reviewed

Bepridil is used to treat angina pectoris (a heart condition characterized by chest pain) among other uses. As with the other drugs in its class, this family of drugs has been found to impact the growth and development of the embryo and should be used cautiously in pregnant women.

Bepridil is absorbed by the body, takes a long time to clear, and the potency of bepridil increases the danger to the breastfeeding infant. Caution is suggested if used by a breastfeeding mother.

Relative infant dose:
Time to clear: Between 7 and 9 days
Lactation risk category: L4
Pregnancy risk category: C
Adult dose: 300 milligrams daily
Alternatives: Nifedipine, Nimodipine

BETAMETHASONE

Trade names: Betameth, Celextone, Betadermetnesol,
Celestone, Diprolene, Dipr, Betnovate, Betnelan,
Diprosone

AAP recommendation: Not reviewed

Betamethasone is a steroid used to reduce inflammation. It generally produces less water retention than other steroids. See prednisone.

Relative infant dose:
Time to clear: Between 22.5 and 28 hours
Lactation risk category: L3
Pregnancy risk category: C
Adult dose: 2.4-4.8 milligrams two or three times daily
Alternatives: Prednisone

BETAXOLOL

Trade names: Kerlone, Betoptic

AAP recommendation: Not reviewed

Betaxolol comes as an eye solution and is used to treat ocular hypertension and glaucoma (abnormally high pressure of the fluid in the eyes). There is only one report about the transfer of betaxolol into breastmilk. It is from the manufacturer and described side effects in one nursing infant. Many drugs in the same class transfer into breastmilk (see atenolol, acebutolol). The manufacturer stated that the amount of betaxolol secreted into breastmilk is high enough to produce side effects in the infant. Caution is urged.

Relative infant dose:
Time to clear: Between 2.5 and 4.5 days
Lactation risk category: L3
Pregnancy risk category: C
Adult dose: 10 milligrams daily
Alternatives:

BETHANECHOL CHLORIDE

Trade names: Urabeth, Urecholine, Urocarb, Myotonine

AAP recommendation: Not reviewed

Bethanechol is used to treat urinary retention (holding urine in the bladder) among other uses. Although bethanechol is poorly absorbed by the body, there are no reports on the transfer of bethanechol into breastmilk. Bethanechol can cause abdominal cramps, colicky pain, nausea, salivation (production of saliva), bronchial constriction (narrowing of breathing tube), and/or diarrhea in infants. There are several reports of discomfort in breastfeeding infants when used directly in infants. It should be used with caution in breastfeeding mothers.

Relative infant dose:
Time to clear: Between 4 and 10 hours
Lactation risk category: L4
Pregnancy risk category: C
Adult dose: 10-50 milligrams two to four times daily
Alternatives:

BISACODYL

Trade names: Bisacodyl, Dacodyl, Dulcolax, Laxit,
Durolax, Apo-Bisacodyl, Bisalax, Paxolax

AAP recommendation: Not reviewed

Bisacodyl is a laxative. It is only transferred into breastmilk in limited amounts because very little is absorbed when taken orally. There are few or no known harmful effects in breastfed infants.

Relative infant dose:
Time to clear:
Lactation risk category: L2
Pregnancy risk category: C
Adult dose: 10-15 milligrams daily
Alternatives:

BISMUTH SUBSALICYLATE

Trade names: Pepto-Bismol

AAP recommendation: Drug whose effect on nursing infants is
unknown but may be of concern

Bismuth subsalicylate is present in many diarrhea mixtures. In contrast to bismuth which is poorly absorbed by the body, salicylate can be absorbed by the body from the diarrhea mixtures. Since salicylates are linked to Reye's syndrome (see aspirin), bismuth subsalicylate should not be used in children in normal cases. Some forms (Parepectolin, Infantol Pink) may contain tincture of opium (morphine).

Relative infant dose:
Time to clear:
Lactation risk category: L3
Pregnancy risk category: C during 1st trimester
D during 2nd and 3rd trimester
Adult dose: 0.524-2.096 grams daily
Alternatives:

BISOPROLOL

Trade names: Ziac, Zebeta, Amizide, Dichlotride, Emcor, Monocor

AAP recommendation: Not reviewed

Bisoprolol is used to treat hypertension (high blood pressure). The manufacturer states that small amounts of bisoprolol are secreted into breastmilk. Other drugs in the same class as bisoprolol are known to produce problems in breastfeeding infants (see atenolol, acebutolol). Ziac combines bisoprolol and hydrochlorothiazide.

Relative infant dose:
Time to clear: Between 1.5 and 2.5 days
Lactation risk category: L3
Pregnancy risk category: C
Adult dose: 5-10 milligrams daily
Alternatives: Propranolol, Metoprolol

BLACK COHOSH

Common names: Baneberry, Black Snakeroot, Bugbane, Squawroot, Rattle root

AAP recommendation: Not reviewed

The roots and stems of this herb are used to treat dysmenorrhea (painful menstration), dyspepsia (digestive function disorder characterized by heartburn, nausea or discomfort), rheumatism (disorder of the connective tissues, muscles or joints which present with pain), as an antitussive to relieve or suppress coughing, and in postmenopausal women as hormone replacement therapy.

This product should not be used in pregnant women. There are no reports on the transfer of black cohosh into breastmilk. However, due to its effect on hormones (estrogen activity), it might lower milk production, but this is not known at this time. Caution is suggested in breastfeeding mothers.

Relative infant dose:
Time to clear:
Lactation risk category: L4
Pregnancy risk category: X
Adult dose:

Alternatives:

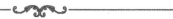

BLESSED THISTLE

Common names: Blessed Thistle

AAP recommendation: Not reviewed

Blessed thistle is believed to be useful for diarrhea, hemorrhage, and fevers. It is thought to be a cough expectorant and to possess other antiseptic properties, among other uses.   Traditionally, it has been used for loss of appetite, gas, cough and congestion, gangrenous ulcers, and dyspepsia. While it is commonly used to increase milk supply, there are no reports that suggest this use.   It is virtually nontoxic.   There are only a few reports that suggest high doses may cause GI symptoms.

Relative infant dose:
Time to clear:
Lactation risk category: L3
Pregnancy risk category:
Adult dose:
Alternatives:

BLUE COHOSH

Common names: Blue ginseng, Squaw root, Papoose root,
                    Yellow ginseng

AAP recommendation: Not reviewed

Blue Cohosh, also known as blue ginseng, squaw root, papoose root or yellow ginseng, is mainly used to start uterine contractions prior to delivery. There is a report of an infant, born to a mother who took blue cohosh 3 weeks prior to delivery, who suffered from severe cardiogenic shock and congestive heart failure. Other studies have shown it to be toxic to the heart. This product should not be used in pregnant women. There are no reports on its transfer into breastmilk, but it is far too dangerous to use in breastfeeding mothers.

Relative infant dose:
Time to clear:
Lactation risk category: L5
Pregnancy risk category: X
Adult dose:

Alternatives:

BROMPHENIRAMINE

Trade names: Dimetane, Brombay, Dimetapp, Bromfed, Dimotane

AAP recommendation: Not reviewed

Brompheniramine is a popular antihistamine used for the relief of nasal or sinus congestion. Although only very small amounts are transferred into breastmilk, there are a number of reported cases of irritability, excessive crying, and sleep disturbances in breastfeeding infants. It should be used with caution in breastfeeding mothers.

Relative infant dose:
Time to clear: Between 4 and 5 days
Lactation risk category: L3
Pregnancy risk category: C
Adult dose: 4 milligrams every 4-6 hours
Alternatives: Loratadine, Cetirizine

BUDESONIDE

Trade names: Rhinocort, Pulmicort Respules, Pulmicort

AAP recommendation: Not reviewed

Budesonide is a steriod used to treat Crohn's disease and as an oral inhalation for the management of asthma and rhinitis (inflammation of the nasal mucous membrane). Only 20% of budesonide taken by a breastfeeding mother is absorbed. If normal doses are used, it is unlikely that amounts large enough to cause side effects would ever reach the milk or be absorbed by the breastfeeding infant.

Relative infant dose:
Time to clear: Between 11 and 14 hours
Lactation risk category: L3
Pregnancy risk category: C
Adult dose: 200-400 micrograms twice daily
Alternatives:

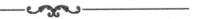

BUPIVACAINE

Trade names: Marcaine, Marcain

AAP recommendation: Not reviewed

Bupivacaine is the most commonly used anesthetic agent during delivery because the amount of bupivacaine that reaches the fetus is the lowest of all the local anesthetics. In one study, it was found that bupivacaine is a safe drug in mothers who plan to breastfeed. In a study of 27 women, the amount of bupivacaine in breastmilk was very low and the dose the infant would receive would be less than 1% of the mothers dose.

Relative infant dose: 1.2%
Time to clear: Between 11 and 13.5 hours
Lactation risk category: L2
Pregnancy risk category: C
Adult dose: One dose of 25-100 milligrams
Alternatives:

BUPRENORPHINE

Trade names: Buprenex, Temgesic, Subutex

AAP recommendation: Not reviewed

Buprenorphine is used for the relief of moderate to severe pain. Buprenorphine may slow the production of milk, although this is not clear. As with most drugs in this class, breastmilk levels are probably low, but long term exposure should be avoided. In one patient who received 4 milligrams per day to help withdraw from other opiates, the amount of buprenorphine transferred by milk was only 3.28 micrograms per day, an amount that is very, very low. As with most opiates, breastmilk levels are probably low, but this drug should not be taken on a long-term basis.

Relative infant dose:
Time to clear: Between 5 hours and 1.5 days
Lactation risk category: L3
Pregnancy risk category: C
Adult dose: 0.3 milligrams every 6 hours as needed
Alternatives:

BUPROPION

Trade names: Wellbutrin, Zyban

AAP recommendation: Drug whose effect on nursing infants is unknown but may be of concern

Bupropion is used as an antidepressant and for smoking cessation therapy. Bupropion may cause birth defects in pregnant women and should not be used in mothers with seizures or infants with seizure disorders. In a recent study of two breastfeeding patients (one took 75 milligrams twice daily and the other took 150 milligrams (sustained release) daily), no bupropion or its by-products were detected in the breastfed infant. Several patients taking bupropion have reported reduced milk supply. This drug is commonly used in breastfeeding mothers without problems, but caution concerning milk supply is suggested.

Relative infant dose: 0.7%
Time to clear: Between 1.5 and 5 days
Lactation risk category: L3
Pregnancy risk category: B
Adult dose: 100 milligrams three times daily
Alternatives: Sertraline, Paroxetine

BUSPIRONE

Trade names: BuSpar, Apo-Buspirone, Novo-Buspirone

AAP recommendation: Not reviewed

Buspirone is used to treat anxiety disorders, sexual dysfunction, and depressive symptoms. There are no reports on the transfer of buspirone into breastmilk. Since buspirone clears the body quickly, it is not likely to build up in the infant's blood. Compared to other drugs in the Valium family, buspirone may be a suitable choice for treatment of anxiety in breastfeeding women.

Relative infant dose:
Time to clear: Between 8 and 15 hours
Lactation risk category: L3
Pregnancy risk category: B
Adult dose: 5 milligrams three times daily
Alternatives:

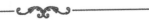

BUTABARBITAL

Trade names: Butisol, Butalan, Ampyrox

AAP recommendation: Not reviewed

Butabarbital is used to sedate patients before an operation and to relieve anxiety. Small amounts of butabarbital are transferred into breastmilk. No harmful effects have been reported. Watch infant for drowsiness and sedation.

Relative infant dose:
Time to clear: Between 16.5 and 21 days
Lactation risk category: L3
Pregnancy risk category: D
Adult dose: 15-30 milligrams three or four times daily
Alternatives:

BUTORPHANOL

Trade names: Stadol

AAP recommendation: Maternal medication usually compatible with breastfeeding

Butorphanol is used to treat moderate to severe pain associated with delivery, cancer, burns, etc. It is available as an injection or a nasal spray. Butorphanol has been found to produce an unusual fetal heart rate pattern and distress in the infant and hallucinogenic-like responses in postpartum women (< 3%). It is transferred into breastmilk in low to moderate levels. However, the levels attained in an infant are considered very low to insignificant.

Relative infant dose: 0.5%
Time to clear: Between 12 and 20 hours
Lactation risk category: L3
Pregnancy risk category: B during 1st and 2nd trimester
D during 3rd trimester
Adult dose: 1-4 milligrams injected into the muscle every 3-4 hours OR
0.5-2 milligrams intravenously every 3-4 hours
Alternatives:

CABERGOLINE

Trade names: Dostinex

AAP recommendation: Not reviewed

Cabergoline is used for disorders that present with high prolactin levels, such as pituitary tumors. In many countries, cabergoline is used to stop breastmilk production with just 2 doses. The transfer of cabergoline into breastmilk has not been reported, but it is probably quite low. In patients with exceedingly high prolactin levels who receive cabergoline and wish to breastfeed, the dose of cabergoline used in the mother can be lowered so that prolactin levels are reduced to a safe range, but still high enough to support breastmilk production (100-200 nanograms per milliliter).

Relative infant dose:
Time to clear: Between 13.5 and 16.5 days
Lactation risk category: L4
Pregnancy risk category: B
Adult dose: 0.25-1 milligram twice a week
Alternatives:

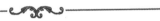

CAFFEINE

Trade names: Vivarin, Nodoz, Coffee

AAP recommendation: Maternal medication usually compatible with breastfeeding

Caffeine is a naturally occurring compound present in many foods and drinks (coffee, tea, and soft drinks). There is some evidence that long-term coffee drinking may reduce the iron content of breastmilk. Irritability and insomnia may occur and have been reported in breastfed infants. Occasional use of caffeine is not a problem, but heavy, daily use may lead to high levels in the younger breastfeeding infant. By 9 months, most infants are able to clear caffeine from their systems as quickly as adults.

Relative infant dose: 6.0%
Time to clear: Between 19.5 and 24.5 hours
Lactation risk category: L2
Pregnancy risk category: B
Adult dose:
Alternatives:

CALCIPOTRIENE

Trade names: Dovonex

AAP recommendation: Not reviewed

Calcipotriene comes in a cream, ointment or solution to be applied to affected psoriasis areas (reddish, silvery-scaled lesions which occur mainly on the elbows, knees, scalp and trunk). Only 5-6% is absorbed by the body when calcipotriene is applied on the skin. Less than 1% is absorbed when the solution is applied to the scalp. However, if calcipotriene is used over wide areas of the body, it is possible that a large amount could be absorbed; although, this is unlikely. If calcipotriene is applied to a small area of the body, it is unlikely to cause increased blood levels. In this case, there will be little to none in the breastmilk.

Relative infant dose:
Time to clear:
Lactation risk category: L3
Pregnancy risk category: C
Adult dose: Apply to skin lesions twice daily
Alternatives:

CALCITRIOL

Trade names: Rocaltrol

AAP recommendation: Not reviewed

Calcitriol (vitamin D analog) is used to treat hypocalcemia (low blood levels of calcium) in patients undergoing renal dialysis and renal osteodystrophy (defective bone development). It is not likely that normal amounts of calcitriol would lead to levels in breastmilk that would cause problems in breastfeeding infants. Some caution is recommended.

Relative infant dose:
Time to clear: Between 20 hours and 1.5 days
Lactation risk category: L3
Pregnancy risk category: C
Adult dose: Variable, but 0.25-0.5 micrograms per day initially
Alternatives: Vitamin D

CALENDULA

Trade names: Calendula, Marigold, Garden Marigold, Holligold, Gold Bloom, Marybud

AAP recommendation: Not reviewed

Calendula, grown worldwide, has been used to stimulate wound healing, treat conjunctivitis (pink eye) and other inflammations of the eye, as an anti-inflammatory, and lastly to relieve or prevent spasms. Despite these claims, there are almost no studies that show that calendula cures any of these disorders. There are also no reports of harmful side effects, with the exception of allergies.

Relative infant dose:
Time to clear:
Lactation risk category: L3
Pregnancy risk category:
Adult dose:
Alternatives:

CANDESARTAN

Trade names: Atacand

AAP recommendation: Not reviewed

Candesartan is used to treat hypertension (high blood pressure), kidney damage in diabetics, and congestive heart failure. This family of drugs should not be taken during the second and third trimesters of pregnancy as they may cause extremely low blood pressure, under-development of the fetal skull, irreversible renal failure, and death of the newborn infant. However, there are no reports on the transfer of candesartan into breastmilk. Some caution is suggested in the newborn period. This drug should be used with caution in breastfeeding mothers of premature infants.

Relative infant dose:
Time to clear: Between 36 and 45 hours
Lactation risk category: L4
Pregnancy risk category: D
Adult dose: 4-32 milligrams daily
Alternatives: Captopril, Enalapril

CANNABIS

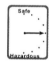

Common names: Marijuana

AAP recommendation: Contraindicated by the American Academy of Pediatrics in breastfeeding mothers

Cannibis is commonly known as marijuana. It has been reported that small to moderate amounts of marijuana transfer into breastmilk. Marijuana can cause sedation and growth delay in large doses. In one study of 27 women who smoked marijuana during breastfeeding, no differences were noted in outcomes of growth, mental, and motor development. Infants will test positive in drug screens for days to weeks following exposure to marijuana in breastmilk. Legal consequences could occur.

Relative infant dose:
Time to clear: Between 4 and 12 days
Lactation risk category: L5
Pregnancy risk category: C
Adult dose:
Alternatives:

CAPSAICIN

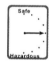

Trade names: Zostrix, Axsain, Capsin, Capzasin-P, Capsig, No-Pain, Absorbine Jr. Arthritis, Arthricare, Natraflex

AAP recommendation: Not reviewed

Capsaicin comes from red peppers and is applied on the skin for pain relief. There are no reports on the transfer of capsaicin into breastmilk. Mothers should not apply capsaicin to the nipple or areola unless it is thoroughly removed before breastfeeding. Be sure to wash hands thoroughly after application to avoid transfer to the infant.

Relative infant dose:
Time to clear:
Lactation risk category: L3
Pregnancy risk category: C
Adult dose:
Alternatives:

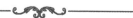

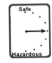

CAPTOPRIL

Trade names: Capoten, Apo-Capto, Acenorm, Enzace,
Novo-Captopril, Acepril

AAP recommendation: Maternal medication usually compatible with
breastfeeding

Captopril is mainly used to treat high blood pressure and is transferred into breastmilk in small amounts. No harmful effects have been reported in the breastfeeding infant. However, the infant should be observed for low blood pressure. Captopril should only be used if its continued use is important for the mother's health.

Relative infant dose: 0.02%
Time to clear: Between 8.8 and 11 hours
Lactation risk category: L3
Pregnancy risk category: D
Adult dose: 50 milligrams three times daily
Alternatives: Enalapril

CARBAMAZEPINE

Trade names: Tegretol, Epitol, Carbatrol, Mazepine, Teril

AAP recommendation: Maternal medication usually compatible with
breastfeeding

Carbamazepine is used to treat epilepsy (convulsions) and depression, among other uses. Carbamazepine is transferred into breastmilk in low levels. No adverse effects have been noted in the breastfeeding infant because the amount of carbamazepine that is transferred into breastmilk is quite low. It is one of the most commonly used anticonvulsants in pediatric patients. Observe for sedative effects in the breastfed infant.

Relative infant dose: 4.4%
Time to clear: Between 3 and 11.5 days
Lactation risk category: L2
Pregnancy risk category: C
Adult dose: 800-1200 milligrams in divided doses three or four times
daily
Alternatives:

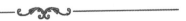

CARBENICILLIN

Trade names: Geopen, Geocillin, Carindacillin, Carbapen
AAP recommendation: Not reviewed

Carbenicillin is used as an antibiotic against upper and lower urinary tract infections and prostatitis. Only limited amounts of carbenicillin are transferred into breastmilk. Due to the poor oral absorption of carbenicillin, the amount absorbed by a breastfeeding infant would be very small. Observe for changes in stool patterns such as diarrhea.

Relative infant dose: 0.3%
Time to clear: Between 4 and 5 hours
Lactation risk category: L1
Pregnancy risk category: B
Adult dose: 382-764 milligrams every 6 hours
Alternatives:

CARTEOLOL

Trade names: Cartrol, Teoptic
AAP recommendation: Not reviewed

Carteolol is a beta blocker used to treat high blood pressure. There are no reports on the transfer of carteolol into breastmilk. Some caution is recommended, however. Observe for weakness, sedation, poor feeding in the infant.

Relative infant dose:
Time to clear: Between 24 and 30 hours
Lactation risk category: L3
Pregnancy risk category: C
Adult dose: 2.5-5 milligrams daily
Alternatives: Propranolol, Metoprolol

CARVEDILOL

Trade names: Coreg, Eucardic, Proreg, Dilatrend
AAP recommendation: Not reviewed

Carvedilol is used to treat high blood pressure and congestive heart failure. There are no reports on the transfer of carvedilol in breastmilk. However, based on its chemical structure, some of the drug might transfer to breastmilk. Caution is generally recommended with all the drugs in this class until we have reports on the levels in breastmilk.

Relative infant dose:
Time to clear: Between 28 and 50 hours
Lactation risk category: L3
Pregnancy risk category: C
Adult dose: 6.25-12.5 milligrams twice daily
Alternatives: Propranolol, Metoprolol.

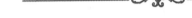

CASCARA SAGRADA

Trade names:
AAP recommendation: Maternal medication usually compatible with breastfeeding

Cascara sagrada is used as a laxative. Very small amounts are transferred into breastmilk; although, exact amounts have not been published. Cascara sagrada might cause loose stools and diarrhea in breastfeeding newborns.

Relative infant dose:
Time to clear:
Lactation risk category: L3
Pregnancy risk category: C
Adult dose: 5 milliliters daily
Alternatives:

CASTOR OIL

Trade names: Alphamul, Neoloid, Emulsoil, Seda-rash, Exzem Oil
AAP recommendation: Not reviewed

Castor oil is prepared from the bean of the castor plant and is a laxative. The transfer of castor oil into breastmilk is unknown. Large amounts could possibly produce diarrhea, insomnia (sleeplessness) and tremors in breastfeeding infants. Caution should be used.

Relative infant dose:
Time to clear:

Lactation risk category: L3
Pregnancy risk category: X
Adult dose:
Alternatives:

CEFADROXIL

Trade names: Ultracef, Duricef, Baxan

AAP recommendation: Maternal medication usually compatible with breastfeeding

Cefadroxil is an antibiotic. Only small amounts are known to be secreted into breastmilk. Observe breastfeeding infant for diarrhea.

Relative infant dose: 1.3%
Time to clear: Between 6 and 7.5 hours
Lactation risk category: L1
Pregnancy risk category: B
Adult dose: 0.5-1 gram twice daily
Alternatives:

CEFAZOLIN

Trade names: Ancef, Kefzol, Cefamezin

AAP recommendation: Maternal medication usually compatible with breastfeeding

Cefazolin is an antibiotic and is minimally transferred into breastmilk. Because it is poorly absorbed, the breastfeeding infant would only be exposed to a very small amount of cefazolin. Blood levels in infants are reported to be too small to be detected.

Relative infant dose: 0.8%
Time to clear: Between 5 and 11 hours
Lactation risk category: L1
Pregnancy risk category: B
Adult dose: 250-2000 milligrams three times daily
Alternatives:

CEFDINIR

Trade names: Omnicef

AAP recommendation: Not reviewed

Cefdinir is an antibiotic. Following administration of a 600 milligram oral dose, no cefdinir was detected in breastmilk.

Relative infant dose:
Time to clear: Between 7 and 8.5 hours
Lactation risk category: L2
Pregnancy risk category: B
Adult dose: 14 milligrams per kilogram per day
Alternatives:

CEFEPIME

Trade names: Maxipime

AAP recommendation: Not reviewed

Cefepime is an antibiotic that is transferred into breastmilk in small amounts. However, the amount transferred may be too small to produce any symptoms other than possible changes in gut flora and diarrhea.

Relative infant dose: 0.3%
Time to clear: Between 8 and 10 hours
Lactation risk category: L2
Pregnancy risk category: B
Adult dose: 1-2 grams twice daily
Alternatives:

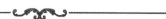

CEFIXIME

Trade names: Suprax

AAP recommendation: Not reviewed

Cefixime is an antibiotic that is transferred into breastmilk to a limited degree. It is poorly absorbed (30-50%) when taken by mouth. In one study of a mother receiving 100 milligrams, it was undetected in her breastmilk from 1-6 hours after the dose.

Relative infant dose:
Time to clear: Between 28 and 35 hours
Lactation risk category: L2
Pregnancy risk category: B
Adult dose: 200 milligrams twice daily
Alternatives:

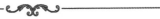

CEFOPERAZONE SODIUM

Trade names: Cefobid, Dicapen

AAP recommendation: Not reviewed

Cefoperazone is an antibiotic, is only available as an injection, and is poorly transferred into breastmilk. Cefoperazone is destroyed in the gastrointestinal tract of a breastfeeding infant, limiting the amount the infant can absorb. It is unlikely that the infant would receive enough cefoperazone to cause side effects.

Relative infant dose: 0.4%
Time to clear: Between 8 and 10 hours.
Lactation risk category: L2
Pregnancy risk category: B
Adult dose: 1-2 grams twice daily
Alternatives:

CEFOTAXIME

Trade names: Claforan

AAP recommendation: Maternal medication usually compatible with breastfeeding

Cefotaxime is an antibiotic that is minimally transferred into breastmilk. However, no effects on breastfeeding infants have been noted. In a group of 2-3 mothers receiving 1000 milligrams intravenously, none to trace amounts were found in milk after 6 hours.

Relative infant dose: 0.3%
Time to clear: Between 3 and 3.5 hours
Lactation risk category: L2
Pregnancy risk category: B
Adult dose: 1-2 grams every 12 hours

Alternatives:

CEFOXITIN

Trade names: Mefoxin

AAP recommendation: Maternal medication usually compatible with breastfeeding

Cefoxitin is an antibiotic that is transferred into breastmilk in very low levels. In a study of 18 women receiving 2000-4000 milligrams doses, only one breastmilk sample contained cefoxitin (0.9 milligrams per liter). The levels in the other mothers' milk were too low to be detected.

Relative infant dose: 0.2%
Time to clear: Between 3 and 5.5 hours
Lactation risk category: L1
Pregnancy risk category: B
Adult dose: 1-2 grams three times daily
Alternatives:

CEFPROZIL

Trade names: Cefzil

AAP recommendation: Maternal medication usually compatible with breastfeeding

Cefprozil is an antibiotic that is transferred into breastmilk in low levels. The levels are so low it is unlikely an infant would ingest enough to produce a harmful effect.

Relative infant dose: 3.6%
Time to clear: Between 5 and 6.5 hours
Lactation risk category: L1
Pregnancy risk category: C
Adult dose: 250 milligrams twice daily
Alternatives:

CEFTRIAXONE

Trade names: Rocephin

AAP recommendation: Maternal medication usually compatible with breastfeeding

Ceftriaxone is an antibiotic commonly used in infants. Small amounts of ceftriaxone are transferred into breastmilk. Because ceftriaxone is poorly absorbed after it is taken by mouth, only very small amounts will be absorbed by the infant from breastmilk. No harmful effects were noted even when a breastfeeding mother took high doses of ceftriaxone. Observe infant for diarrhea or blood in the stools.

Relative infant dose: 4.2%
Time to clear: Between 29 and 36.5 hours
Lactation risk category: L2
Pregnancy risk category: B
Adult dose: 1-2 grams once to twice daily
Alternatives:

CEFUROXIME

Trade names: Ceftin, Zinacef, Kefurox, Zinnat

AAP recommendation: Not reviewed

Cefuroxime is an antibiotic that can be taken by mouth or as an injection. The manufacturer states that it is secreted into breastmilk in small amounts, but the levels are not known. So far, no harmful effects in infants have been reported. It is commonly used in infants and children.

Relative infant dose:
Time to clear: Between 5.5 and 7 hours
Lactation risk category: L2
Pregnancy risk category: B
Adult dose: 250-500 milligrams twice daily
Alternatives:

CELECOXIB

Trade names: Celebrex

AAP recommendation: Not reviewed

Celecoxib is an anti-inflammatory drug used to treat painful menstruation, osteoarthritis (breakdown of cartilage in joints), rheumatoid arthritis, and pain. Milk levels of celecoxib are very low. Blood levels of celecoxib in two breastfeeding infants were undetectable.

Relative infant dose: 0.3%
Time to clear: Between 45 and 56 hours
Lactation risk category: L2
Pregnancy risk category: C
Adult dose: 100-400 milligrams daily
Alternatives: Ibuprofen

CEPHALEXIN

Trade names: Keflex, Ceporex, Novo-Lexin, Ibilex

AAP recommendation: Not reviewed

Cephalexin is an antibiotic. Only minimal amounts are secreted into breastmilk, which are probably too low to cause problems in the infant. It is commonly used for mastitis in breastfeeding women.

Relative infant dose: 0.5%
Time to clear: Between 3.5 and 6.5 hours
Lactation risk category: L1
Pregnancy risk category: B
Adult dose: 250-1000 milligrams every 6 hours
Alternatives:

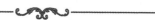

CETIRIZINE

Trade names: Zyrtec, Zirtek

AAP recommendation: Not reviewed

Cetirizine is an antihistamine useful for seasonal allergic rhinitis (inflammation of the nasal mucous membranes). It produces minimal sedation. While we do not know the exact levels in milk, a very small amount of cetirizine probably transfers into breastmilk. It is commonly used in breastfeeding mothers and even young children.

Relative infant dose:
Time to clear: Between 33 and 41.5 hours
Lactation risk category: L2
Pregnancy risk category: B
Adult dose: 5-10 milligrams daily
Alternatives:

CHAMOMILE, GERMAN

Common names: Hungarian Chamomile, Sweet False, Wild Chamomile

AAP recommendation: Not reviewed

Chamomile is mainly used for its anti-inflammatory, carminative (helps to expel gas from the intestinal tract), antispasmodic (relieves or prevents spasms), mild sedative (sleeping aid), and antiseptic (disinfectant) properties. Several cases of allergic reactions to chamomile have been reported. Asthmatics and pregnant and lactating women should avoid this product. However, aside from allergies, chamomile is probably safe for use in breastfeeding mothers.

Relative infant dose:
Time to clear:
Lactation risk category: L3
Pregnancy risk category:
Adult dose:
Alternatives:

CHLORHEXIDINE

Trade names: Peridex, Bactoshield, Betasept, Dyna-hex, Hexol, Hibiclens, Hibitane, Savlon, Bactigras

AAP recommendation: Not reviewed

Chlorhexidine is available as an oral rinse and as lozenges. It is also available as a liquid to disinfect the skin. Chlorhexidine is poorly absorbed by the body and is not likely to cause harmful effects in breastfeeding infants.

Relative infant dose:

Time to clear:	Between 16 and 20 hours
Lactation risk category:	L2
Pregnancy risk category:	B
Adult dose:	
Alternatives:	

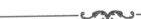

CHLOROTHIAZIDE

Trade names: Hydrodiuril, Chlotride, Saluric

AAP recommendation: Maternal medication usually compatible with breastfeeding

Chlorothiazide is a diuretic (increases the flow of urine) and is used to treat high blood pressure. Most diuretics in the same class as chlorothiazide are okay to take when breastfeeding if the dosage is low and the mother's milk supply is watched closely to make sure it does not decrease.

Relative infant dose:	2.1%
Time to clear:	Between 6 and 7.5 hours
Lactation risk category:	L3
Pregnancy risk category:	D
Adult dose:	500-2000 milligrams every 12-24 hours
Alternatives:	

CHLORPHENIRAMINE

Trade names: Aller-chlor, Chlor-Tripolon, Chlor-Trimeton, Demazin, Alunex, Piridon

AAP recommendation: Not reviewed

Chlorpheniramine is a commonly used antihistamine in over-the-counter remedies. Although there are no reports on its transfer into breastmilk, there are also no reports on harmful effects in infants. Sedation is the only likely side effect.

Relative infant dose:	
Time to clear:	Between 2 and 9 days
Lactation risk category:	L3
Pregnancy risk category:	B
Adult dose:	4 milligrams every 4-6 hours
Alternatives:	Cetirizine, Loratadine

CHLORPROPAMIDE

Trade names: Diabenese, Novopropamide, Melitase

AAP recommendation: Drug whose effect on nursing infants is
unknown but may be of concern

Chlorpropamide is used in the management of Type 2 diabetes mellitus and is transferred into breastmilk, although the levels are low. It could potentially cause hypoglycemia (low blood sugar) in breastfeeding infants; although, effects are largely unknown and unreported.

Relative infant dose: 10.5%
Time to clear: Between 5.5 and 7 days
Lactation risk category: L3
Pregnancy risk category: D
Adult dose: 250-500 milligrams daily
Alternatives:

CHOLESTYRAMINE

Trade names: Questran, Cholybar, Novo-Cholamine

AAP recommendation: Not reviewed

Cholestyramine is used to treat hypercholersterolemia (high cholesterol) among other uses. Cholestryramine is not absorbed by the body and does not transfer into breastmilk.

Relative infant dose:
Time to clear:
Lactation risk category: L1
Pregnancy risk category: C
Adult dose: 16-32 grams per day
Alternatives:

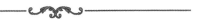

CHONDROITIN SULFATE

Trade names: Viscoat

AAP recommendation: Not reviewed

Chondroitin comes from natural sources such as shark or cow cartilage. So far, chondroitin has been found to be nontoxic. Chondroitin is not likely to transfer into breastmilk due to its structure. It is also poorly absorbed by the body when taken by mouth and is, therefore, unlikely to pose a problem for a breastfeeding infant.

Relative infant dose:
Time to clear:
Lactation risk category: L3
Pregnancy risk category:
Adult dose:
Alternatives:

CIMETIDINE

Trade names: Tagamet, Magicul, Sigmetadine, Peptimax, Zita

AAP recommendation: Maternal medication usually compatible with breastfeeding

Cimetidine is used as short-term treatment of duodenal (small intestine) and gastric (stomach) ulcers, among other uses. Cimetidine is transferred into breastmilk, but the levels are too low to produce problems in an infant. Even though cimetidine transfers into human milk, there are much better choices. It is okay to use when breastfeeding if it is only used for a few days. Omeprazole, famotidine and nizatidine are better alternatives.

Relative infant dose: 32.6%
Time to clear: Between 8 and 10 hours
Lactation risk category: L2
Pregnancy risk category: B
Adult dose: 800 milligrams at bedtime
Alternatives: Famotidine, Nizatidine

CIPROFLOXACIN

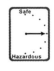

Trade names: Cipro, Ciloxan, Ciproxin

AAP recommendation: Maternal medication usually compatible with breastfeeding

Ciprofloxacin is an antibiotic that is presently the drug of choice to prevent and treat anthrax, common urinary tract infections, and gut infections. The levels of ciprofloxacin in breastmilk conflict in the reports and vary from low to moderate. Current studies seem to suggest that the amount of ciprofloxacin present in milk is quite low. Ciprofloxacin is also available in several ophthalmic (eye) preparations like Ciloxan. Used in the eye, the dose in a nursing mother would be very small. The eye preparations would be okay for breastfeeding mothers. Ciprofloxacin is approved by the AAP (American Academy of Pediatrics) for use in breastfeeding women. Observe for bloody diarrhea in the infant, although this is rare.

Relative infant dose:	2.7%
Time to clear:	Between 16.5 and 20.5 hours
Lactation risk category:	L3
Pregnancy risk category:	C
Adult dose:	250 milligrams twice daily
Alternatives:	Norfloxacin, Ofloxacin

CITALOPRAM

Trade names: Celexa, Cipramil, Talam, Talohexal

AAP recommendation: Not reviewed

Citalopram is an antidepressant. Its effects are somewhat similar to Prozac (fluoxetine) and Zoloft (sertraline). Citalopram is transferred into breastmilk in low to moderate levels. Depending on the amount of citalopram the mother takes, the breastfeeding infant may have an 'uneasy' sleep pattern, extreme sedation, or, as in several studies, no effects at all. The manufacturer reports several cases of sedation in breastfed infants. This author has received several case reports of sedation as well. Citalopram should be used cautiously in newborns and infants less than 2 months of age. See sertraline as alternative.

Relative infant dose:	3.6%
Time to clear:	Between 6 and 7.5 days
Lactation risk category:	L3
Pregnancy risk category:	C
Adult dose:	20-40 milligrams daily
Alternatives:	Sertraline, Paxil

CLARITHROMYCIN

Trade names: Biaxin, Klacid, Klaricid

AAP recommendation: Not reviewed

Clarithromycin is an antibiotic. No studies have been performed on the transfer of clarithromycin into breastmilk. Clarithromycin is probably transferred into milk in low levels. However, it is a commonly used pediatric antibiotic in infants older than 6 months. Clarithromycin is probably quite safe for a breastfeeding mother. However, see azithromycin as an alternative.

Relative infant dose:
Time to clear: Between 20 and 35 hours
Lactation risk category: L2
Pregnancy risk category: C
Adult dose: 250 milligrams twice daily
Alternatives:

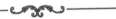

CLEMASTINE

Trade names: Tavist, Tavegyl

AAP recommendation: Drug associated with significant side effects and should be taken with caution

Clemastine is a long-acting antihistamine. Clemastine is transferred into breastmilk and may cause drowsiness, irritability, refusal to feed, and neck stiffness in the breastfeeding infant. Some caution is recommended.

Relative infant dose: 5.2%
Time to clear: Between 1.5 and 2.5 days
Lactation risk category: L4
Pregnancy risk category: C
Adult dose: 1.34 to 2.68 milligrams two or three times daily
Alternatives: Cetirazine, Loratadine

CLINDAMYCIN

Trade names: Cleocin, Clindatech, Dalacin

AAP recommendation: Maternal medication usually compatible with breastfeeding

Clindamycin is an antibiotic used orally, by injection, and topically on the skin. Clindamycin is transferred into breastmilk, but only in small amounts (about 1.6% of the mother's dose). Changes in gastrointestinal flora are possible even though the dose is low. One case of bloody stools (pseudomembranous colitis) has been associated with clindamycin and gentamycin therapy.

However, clindamycin is a popular antibiotic for severe infections in infants and children and is commonly used. It is increasingly being used for resistant staph infections and is probably safe for breastfeeding mothers.

Relative infant dose: 1.7%
Time to clear: Between 11.5 and 14.5 hours
Lactation risk category: L3
Pregnancy risk category: B
Adult dose: 150-450 milligrams every 6 hours
Alternatives:

CLOMIPHENE

Trade names: Clomid, Serophene, Milophene
AAP recommendation: Not reviewed

Clomiphene is used to treat ovarian failure in infertile women. Clomiphene appears to be very effective in stopping breastmilk production when used less than 4 days postpartum. It is believed to have very little effect on milk production after lactation is well established. We do not know how much transfers into milk, but it is unlikely to produce an effect in a breastfeeding infant.

Relative infant dose:
Time to clear: Between 20 and 35 days
Lactation risk category: L4
Pregnancy risk category: X
Adult dose: 50 milligrams daily
Alternatives:

CLONAZEPAM

Trade names: Klonopin, Apo-Clonazepam, Rivotril,
                Paxam, PMS-Clonazepam
AAP recommendation: Not reviewed

Clonazepam is used as an anticonvulsant. It is transferred into breastmilk in small amounts. In one infant exposed at birth and during lactation, the infant's blood levels at 14 days were 4 times less than the blood levels at birth, suggesting limited transfer from breastmilk.

Relative infant dose:
Time to clear: Between 3 and 10.5 days

Lactation risk category: L3
Pregnancy risk category: C
Adult dose: 0.5-1 milligram three times daily
Alternatives:

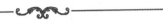

CLONIDINE

Trade names: Catapres, Dixarit, Apo-Clonidine,
Novo-Clonidine

AAP recommendation: Not reviewed

Clonidine is used to treat hypertension (high blood pressure). It is transferred into breastmilk when taken both by mouth and when a mother uses a clonidine skin patch. Symptoms of harmful effects in the newborn are unreported and are unlikely in normal full term infants. Clonidine may reduce prolactin secretion, possibly reducing milk production if taken right after birth.

Relative infant dose: 7.5%
Time to clear: Between 3.5 and 5 days
Lactation risk category: L3
Pregnancy risk category: C
Adult dose: 0.1-0.3 milligrams twice daily
Alternatives:

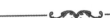

CLOTRIMAZOLE

Trade names: Gyne-Lotrimin, Mycelex, Lotrimin,
FemCare, Trivaqizole, Clotrimaderm, Myclo, Canesten,
Clonea, Hiderm

AAP recommendation: Not reviewed

Clotrimazole is an antifungal agent that comes as oral lozenges, topical creams, intravaginal tablets, and creams. There are no reports on the transfer of clotrimazole into breastmilk. However, when inserted into the vagina, only 3-10% of the drug is absorbed. It seems unlikely that levels absorbed by a breastfeeding infant would be high enough to produce harmful effects. Clotrimazole is commonly applied on the skin to treat fungal (yeast) infections. However, it is known to cause contact dermatitis on skin and nipples and should not be used directly on a mother's nipple and areola. Use miconazole instead.

Relative infant dose:

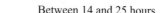

Time to clear: Between 14 and 25 hours
Lactation risk category: L1
Pregnancy risk category: B during 1st and 2nd trimester
C during 3rd trimester
Adult dose: 500 milligrams intravaginally at bedtime
Alternatives: Fluconazole, Miconazole

CLOXACILLIN

Trade names: Tegopen, Cloxapen, Novo-Cloxin, Orbenin, Alclox, Kloxerate-DC

AAP recommendation: Not reviewed

Cloxacillin is a penicillin antibiotic. It is transferred into breastmilk, but, as with most penicillins, it is unlikely the levels would cause problems in the breastfeeding infant. Watch for diarrhea in the infant.

Relative infant dose: 0.2%
Time to clear: Between 3 and 15 hours
Lactation risk category: L2
Pregnancy risk category: B
Adult dose: 250-500 milligrams every 6 hours
Alternatives:

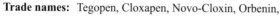

COCAINE

Common names: Crack

AAP recommendation: Contraindicated by the American Academy of Pediatrics in breastfeeding mothers

Cocaine is a powerful stimulant as well as a local anesthetic. It is well absorbed from all locations including the stomach, nasal passages and the lung following inhalation. Even after the effects of cocaine are gone, breastmilk may still contain large amounts of benzoylecgonine, the break down product (metabolite) of cocaine. Thus, breastfeeding infants will test positive for cocaine with a urine test for long periods of time.

Studies of the transfer of cocaine into breastmilk have not been reported, but we suspect large amounts transfer. Excitation in the infant has been reported in breastfeeding mothers who use cocaine. Do not use it topically on the nipples. Breastfeeding mothers should NOT use any manner of cocaine - topical, intranasal, or smoked. If a mother does ingest cocaine, she should pump to maintain her milk supply and discard the milk for 24 hours to allow the active cocaine to clear her system. The infant could still test positive for urine cocaine metabolites for 7 or more days. DO NOT allow anyone to smoke cocaine around the infant as the baby may ingest small amounts of cocaine by inhaling the smoke.

Relative infant dose:
Time to clear: Between 3 and 4 hours
Lactation risk category: L5
Pregnancy risk category: C during 1st and 2nd trimester
X during 3rd trimester

Adult dose:
Alternatives:

CODEINE

Trade names: Empirin #3 # 4, Tylenol # 3 # 4, Penntuss, Actacode, Codalgin, Codral, Panadeine, Veganin, Kaodene, Teropin

AAP recommendation: Maternal medication usually compatible with breastfeeding

Codeine is used to treat mild to moderate pain. The amount of codeine secreted into breastmilk is low and dose dependent. The infant response is higher during the first or second week of life. Four cases of neonatal apnea (breathing temporarily stops) have been reported after the mothers took 60 milligrams codeine every 4-6 hours; although, codeine was not detected in the serum of the infants tested. The apnea stopped when the mother stopped taking codeine. There are few reported side effects following codeine doses of 30 milligrams, and it is believed to produce only very small side effects in newborns. But, observe infants for sedation and poor feeding.

Relative infant dose: 8.0%
Time to clear: Between 11.5 and 14.5 hours
Lactation risk category: L3
Pregnancy risk category: C
Adult dose: 15-60 milligrams every 4-6 hours
Alternatives:

COMFREY

Common names: Russian comfrey, Knitbone, Bruisewort, Blackwort, Slippery root

AAP recommendation: Not reviewed

Comfrey is believed to heal gastric ulcers, hemorrhoids, and suppress bronchial congestion and inflammation, although these claims are poorly supported. A number of significant human side effects have been reported including several deaths - all linked to drinking comfrey tea or yerba mate tea. Comfrey and members of this family are very dangerous and should not be applied to the skin, taken by mouth, or used in any form by breastfeeding mothers. This herb is definitely contraindicated in breastfeeding mothers.

Relative infant dose:
Time to clear:
Lactation risk category: L5
Pregnancy risk category: X
Adult dose:
Alternatives:

CO-TRIMOXAZOLE

Trade names: TMP-SMZ, Bactrim, Cotrim, Septra, Septrin, Respax, Trimogal

AAP recommendation: Maternal medication usually compatible with breastfeeding

Co-trimoxazole is the mixture of trimethoprim and sulfamethoxazole. See the drug entries for each of these products.

Relative infant dose:
Time to clear:
Lactation risk category: L3
Pregnancy risk category:
Adult dose: 160 milligrams twice daily
Alternatives:

CROMOLYN SODIUM

Trade names: Nasalcrom, Gastrocrom, Intal, Nalcrom,
Opticrom, Rhynacrom, Vistacrom, Cromese, Rynacrom

AAP recommendation: Not reviewed

Cromolyn is used as an anti-asthmatic and anti-allergic agent. Although there are no reports on the transfer of cromolyn into breastmilk, almost none would be found in milk. Less than 1% of this drug is absorbed from the mother's (and probably the infant's) gastrointestinal tract, so it is unlikely to produce harmful effects in nursing infants. This drug is frequently used in pediatric patients.

Relative infant dose:
Time to clear: Between 5.5 and 7.5 hours
Lactation risk category: L1
Pregnancy risk category: B
Adult dose: 20 milligrams four times daily via inhalation
Alternatives:

CYCLOBENZAPRINE

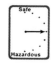

Trade names: Flexeril, Cycoflex, Novo-Cycloprine

AAP recommendation: Not reviewed

Cyclobenzaprine is a muscle relaxant. It is not known if cyclobenzaprine is secreted in breastmilk, but one must assume that its secretion would be similar to the tricyclics antidepressant (see amitriptyline, desipramine) due to its chemical structure. There are no pediatric uses for this drug.

Relative infant dose:
Time to clear: Between 4 and 15 days
Lactation risk category: L3
Pregnancy risk category: B
Adult dose: 20-60 milligrams daily
Alternatives:

CYCLOSPORINE

Trade names: Sandimmune, Neoral, Sandimmun

AAP recommendation: Cytotoxic drug that may interfere with cellular metabolism of the nursing infant

Cyclosporine is an immunosuppresant used to reduce organ rejection following transplant. Cyclosporin is generally transferred into breastmilk in low levels. Due to its immune suppressant properties, it should be used very cautiously in breastfeeding mothers. Most studies suggest levels transferred to the infant are extremely low, but one study found rather high cyclosporine levels in one infant. While no harmful effects have been noted in breastfed infants, immune system shut-down followed by infections are possible. Cyclosporine use in breastfeeding mothers should be closely followed by a doctor.

Relative infant dose: 0.5%
Time to clear: Between 22.5 and 28 hours
Lactation risk category: L3
Pregnancy risk category: C
Adult dose: 5-15 milligrams per kilogram daily
Alternatives:

CYPROHEPTADINE

Trade names: Periactin

AAP recommendation: Not reviewed

Cyproheptadine is an antihistamine with sedative (tranquilizing) effects. It has been used to increase appetite in children and for rashes and itching. There are no reports on its transfer into breastmilk.

Relative infant dose:
Time to clear: Between 2.5 and 3.5 days
Lactation risk category: L3
Pregnancy risk category: B
Adult dose: 4 milligrams three to four times daily
Alternatives: Hydroxyzine

CYTOMEGALOVIRUS

Trade names: Human Cytomegalovirus, CMV

AAP recommendation: Not reviewed

Cytomegalovirus (CMV) is one of the family of herpes viruses. Many infants are exposed in utero and in day care centers. CMV is found in the breastmilk of nearly all CMV-positive women. If a pregnant woman becomes positive late in the pregnancy, the infant is less likely to be severely affected. In most infants from CMV-positive mothers, the CMV found in breastmilk is not very dangerous and these mothers can breastfeed successfully. However, infants whose mothers become CMV-positive while breastfeeding may be very susceptible to the CMV in breastmilk. Therefore, breastmilk from CMV positive mothers should never be given to unprotected infants. If a mom is infected with CMV during lactation, she should not breastfeed.

Relative infant dose:
Time to clear:
Lactation risk category:
Pregnancy risk category:
Adult dose:
Alternatives:

DESIPRAMINE

Trade names: Pertofrane, Norpramin, Novo-Desipramine, Pertofran

AAP recommendation: Drug whose effect on nursing infants is unknown but may be of concern

Desipramine is an antidepressant. It is poorly transferred into breastmilk and reported levels in infants are too low to be measured. So far, no harmful effects have been reported in breastfed infants.

Relative infant dose: 1.0%
Time to clear: Between 1 and 12.5 days
Lactation risk category: L2
Pregnancy risk category: C
Adult dose: 100-200 milligrams daily
Alternatives: Amoxapine, Imipramine

DESLORATADINE

Trade names: Clarinex

AAP recommendation: Not reviewed

Desloratadine is used to relieve allergic rhinitis (inflammation of the nasal mucous membrane). Desloratadine is the active break down product (metabolite) of loratidine (Claritin) which is available over-the-counter to relieve allergies. There are no reports on the transfer of desloratadine into breastmilk, but we do have a good report on loratadine. See loratadine. Desloratadine does not make adults sleepy so it is unlikely to make infants sleepy. Pediatric formulations are available. Loratadine (and probably desloratadine) is a preferred antihistamine for use in breastfeeding mothers.

Relative infant dose: 0.03%
Time to clear: Between 4.5 and 5.5 days
Lactation risk category: L2
Pregnancy risk category: C
Adult dose: 5 milligrams daily
Alternatives: Loratadine

DESOGESTREL AND ETHINYL ESTRADIOL

Trade names: Mircette, Cyclessa

AAP recommendation: Not reviewed

Mircette is a somewhat atypical lower-dose estrogen/progestin oral contraceptive (birth control pill). While most birth control pills contain 40 mcg of ethinyl estradiol or more, the reduced level of estrogen in this product may have less of an impact on milk supply than higher dose products. Small amounts of estrogens and progestins are known to pass into breastmilk, but long-term follow-up of children whose mothers used combination hormonal birth control pills while breastfeeding has shown no harmful effects on their infants. Estrogen-containing birth control pills may decrease the quantity and quality of milk production. While this product is lower in estrogen than most, progestin-only birth control pills are still preferred for breastfeeding mothers.

Relative infant dose:
Time to clear:
Lactation risk category: L3
Pregnancy risk category: X
Adult dose:

Alternatives: Norethindrone

DEXAMETHASONE

Trade names: Decadron, AK-Dex, Maxidex

AAP recommendation: Not reviewed

Dexamethasone is a steroid used for chronic (long-term) swelling among other uses. There are no reports on the transfer of dexamethasone into breastmilk; although, it is likely to be similar to prednisone (extremely low transfer). Doses of prednisone as high as 120 milligrams have failed to produce milk levels that might cause problems in infants. This drug is commonly used in pediatrics to treat immune syndromes such as arthritis and acute onset asthma or other bronchoconstrictive diseases. It is not likely that the amount in breastmilk would produce side effects in infants unless used in high doses or for prolonged periods of time.

Relative infant dose:
Time to clear: Between 13 and 16.5 hours
Lactation risk category: L3
Pregnancy risk category: C
Adult dose: 0.5-9 milligrams daily
Alternatives: Prednisone

DEXTROAMPHETAMINE

Trade names: Dexedrine, Amphetamine, Oxydess, Dexten, Adderall, Dexamphetamine

AAP recommendation: Drugs of abuse for which adverse effects have been reported

Dextroamphetamine is used to treat attention-deficit/hyperactivitity disorder (ADHD). Amphetamines are in most situations poorly transferred into breastmilk; although, excitement and insomnia could result. A study reported that a breastfeeding infant was unaffected when the mother took 20 milligrams of mixed amphetamines daily. Some caution is still suggested with amphetamine use in breastfeeding mothers.

Relative infant dose: 1.8%
Time to clear: Between 24 and 40 hours
Lactation risk category: L4
Pregnancy risk category: C

Adult dose: 5-60 milligrams daily
Alternatives:

DEXTROMETHORPHAN

Trade names: DM, Benylin, Delsym, Pertussin, Cosylan,
Robitussin DM, Benylin DM
AAP recommendation: Not reviewed

Dextromethorphan is used in infants and adults to relieve or suppress coughing. It does not have addictive, analgesic or sedative actions and does not cause breathing difficulties at normal doses. It is the safest of the antitussives and is routinely used in children and infants. There are no reports on its transfer into breastmilk. It is very unlikely that enough would transfer into breastmilk to cause problems in a breastfed infant.

Relative infant dose:
Time to clear: Between 16 and 20 hours
Lactation risk category: L1
Pregnancy risk category: C
Adult dose: 10-20 milligrams every 4 hours
Alternatives: Codeine

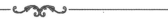

DIAZEPAM

Trade names: Valium, Meval, Novo-Dipam, Vivol,
Antenex, Ducene, Sedapam
AAP recommendation: Drug whose effect on nursing infants is
unknown but may be of concern

Diazepam is used to treat anxiety and convulsive disorders, among other uses. Published reports on milk and plasma levels vary greatly and many are poor studies. The break down product (metabolite) of diazepam, desmethyldiazepam, has a longer half-life and tends to stay in the body for a longer period of time. Some reports of weakness, sedation, and poor suckling have been reported in breastfed infants. If diazepam is used long-term, it could accumulate in the body and increase the risk to the infant. This family, as a rule, is not ideal for breastfeeding mothers due to relatively long half-lives and the development of dependency. However, many newer and shorter-acting benzodiazepines (midazolam, lorazepam, alprazolam) are much safer during lactation provided their use is short-term or used now and then, and in low doses.

Relative infant dose: 9.1%
Time to clear: Between 7 and 9 days
Lactation risk category: L3
L4 if used chronically
Pregnancy risk category: D
Adult dose: 2-10 milligrams two to four times daily
Alternatives: Lorazepam, Midazolam

DIBUCAINE

Trade names: Nupercainal, Cinchocaine, Nupercaine,
Ultraproct, Dermacaine

AAP recommendation: Not reviewed

Dibucaine is a local anesthetic that is applied on the skin. It comes as a cream or ointment. Dibucaine is useful for sunburn, topical burns, rash, rectal hemorrhoids and other skin irritations. Small amounts of dibucaine can be absorbed from irritated skin. There are no reports on the transfer of dibucaine into breastmilk, but it is unlikely to cause problems. Long-term use and use over large areas of the body are discouraged in breastfeeding women. It should not be used on the nipple of a breastfeeding mother.

Relative infant dose:
Time to clear:
Lactation risk category: L3
Pregnancy risk category: C
Adult dose: 10-30 grams daily
Alternatives:

DICLOXACILLIN

Trade names: Pathocil, Dycill, Dynapen, Diclocil,
Dicloxsig

AAP recommendation: Not reviewed

Dicloxacillin is a penicillin antibiotic that is poorly transferred into breastmilk. Dicloxacillin levels were undetectable 6 hours after a mother took an oral dose of 250 milligrams. This penicillin is the most commonly used antibiotic for mastitis in breastfeeding women and has been used safely in millions of breastfeeding mothers. After treatment of mastitis is started, mothers do not need to stop breastfeeding their infants.

Relative infant dose: 1.3%
Time to clear: Between 2.5 and 4 hours
Lactation risk category: L1
Pregnancy risk category: B
Adult dose: 125-250 milligrams every 6 hours
Alternatives:

DIGITOXIN

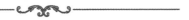

Trade names: Crystodigin

AAP recommendation: Not reviewed

Digitoxin is used to strengthen heart muscle contraction. There are no reports on the transfer of digitoxin into breastmilk. However, some transfer into breastmilk would be expected. Digitoxin is occasionally given to infants. See digoxin.

Relative infant dose:
Time to clear: Between 27 and 33.5 days
Lactation risk category: L3
Pregnancy risk category: C
Adult dose: 0.15 milligrams daily
Alternatives:

DIGOXIN

Trade names: Lanoxin, Lanoxicaps, Novo-Digoxin

AAP recommendation: Maternal medication usually compatible with breastfeeding

Digoxin is used primarily to strengthen the contractile process of the heart. Poor and erratic gastrointestinal absorption of digoxin could theoretically reduce the amount absorbed by the breastfeeding infant. Small amounts of digoxin may transfer into breastmilk, but no problems have been noted in breastfeeding infants.

Relative infant dose: 2.7%
Time to clear: Between 6.5 and 8 days
Lactation risk category: L2
Pregnancy risk category: C
Adult dose: 0.125-0.5 milligrams daily

Alternatives:

DILTIAZEM HCL

Trade names: Cardizem SR, Dilacor-XR, Cardizem CD,
Apo-Diltiazem, Apo-Diltiaz, Cardcal, Coras, Dilzem,
Cardizem, Adizem, Britiazim, Tildiem
AAP recommendation: Maternal medication usually compatible with
breastfeeding

Diltiazem is used orally to treat hypertension (high blood pressure) and angina pectoris (heart cramps), among other uses. Diltiazem is transferred into milk, but the amount is thought to be low. While nifedipine is probably a preferred choice in breastfeeding mothers, the dose of diltiazem transferred to the infant via milk is quite small and is not likely to be a problem.

Relative infant dose: 0.9%
Time to clear: Between 14 and 30 hours
Lactation risk category: L3
Pregnancy risk category: C
Adult dose: 30-90 milligrams four times daily
Alternatives: Nifedipine, Nimodipine, Verapamil

DIMENHYDRINATE

Trade names: Marmine, Dramamine, Traveltabs,
Andrumin, Travacalm

AAP recommendation: Not reviewed

Dimenhydrinate consists of 55% diphenhydramine and 45% of 8-chlorotheophylline. Diphenhydramine (Benadryl) is considered to be the active ingredient. See the monograph for diphenhydramine.

Relative infant dose:
Time to clear: Between 34 and 42.5 hours
Lactation risk category: L2
Pregnancy risk category: B
Adult dose: 50-100 milligrams every 4-6 hours
Alternatives: Cetirizine, Loratadine

DIPHENHYDRAMINE

Trade names: Benadryl, Cheracol, Insomnal, Nytol, Delixir, Paedamin

AAP recommendation: Not reviewed

Diphenhydramine is used to treat allergy symptoms, among other uses. There are no reports on the transfer of diphenhydramine into breastmilk. However, the use of diphenhydramine in breastfeeding mothers is not ideal due to its sedative properties. Non-sedating antihistamines are generally preferred. There are many unsubstantiated reports that diphenhydramine may reduce milk production in some mothers. Mothers should watch their milk supply closely while using this drug, as we have some reports of reduced milk production following the use of Benadryl. Those mothers who already have a poor milk supply should be very cautious.

Relative infant dose:
Time to clear: Between 17 and 21.5 hours
Lactation risk category: L2
Pregnancy risk category: C
Adult dose: 25-50 milligrams three or four times daily
Alternatives: Cetirizine, Loratadine

DIPHENOXYLATE

Trade names: Lomotil, Lofene, Lofenoxal, Tropergen

AAP recommendation: Not reviewed

Lomotil is the combination of diphenoxylate and atropine, and is used to treat diarrhea. Although there are no reports on the transfer of diphenoxylate into breastmilk, it is probably transferred in very small quantities. Some authors think diphenoxylate should not be used in breastfeedng mothers, but this is overly conservative.

Relative infant dose:
Time to clear: Between 10 and 12.5 hours
Lactation risk category: L3
Pregnancy risk category: C
Adult dose: 5 milligrams four times daily
Alternatives:

DIPIVEFRIN

Trade names: AK-Pro, Propine

AAP recommendation: Not reviewed

Dipivefrin is used to treat glaucoma (abnormally high pressure of the fluid in the eyes). It is not known if dipivefrin is transferred into breastmilk, but small amounts may be present. It is unlikely that any dipivefrin present in breastmilk would be absorbed by the infant.

Relative infant dose:
Time to clear:
Lactation risk category: L2
Pregnancy risk category: B
Adult dose: 1 drop in the affected eye every 12 hours
Alternatives:

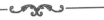

DIRITHROMYCIN

Trade names: Dynabac

AAP recommendation: Not reviewed

Dirithromycin is an antibiotic used to treat lower and upper respiratory tract infections, among other uses. There are no reports on the transfer of dirithromycin, or its metabolite, into breastmilk. Due to the structure of dirithromycin and its distribution largely to tissues, it is unlikely that major levels in breastmilk will result. Alternatives include erythromycin and azithromycin.

Relative infant dose:
Time to clear: Between 3.5 and 10.5 days
Lactation risk category: L3
Pregnancy risk category: C
Adult dose: 500 milligrams daily
Alternatives: Azithromycin, Erythromycin

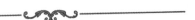

DOCUSATE

Trade names: Colace, Docusate, Softgels, Dialose, Surfak,
Colax-C, Coloxyl, Rectalad, Waxsol, Audinorm,
Diocotyl-medo
AAP recommendation: Not reviewed

Docusate is a stool softener. Although some of the drug is absorbed by the mother via her gastrointestinal tract, transfer into breastmilk is probably minimal. Watch for loose stools or cramping in the infant. It is very likely this drug will cause problems in a breastfeeding infant.

Relative infant dose:
Time to clear:
Lactation risk category: L2
Pregnancy risk category: C
Adult dose: 50-200 milligrams daily
Alternatives:

DORZOLAMIDE

Trade names: Trusopt
AAP recommendation: Not reviewed

Dorzolamide is used in the treatment of glaucoma (abnormally high pressure of the fluid in the eyes). There are no reports on the levels in breastmilk. Transfer of small amounts into breastmilk over a long period could cause problems for breastfeeding infants. Breastfeeding mothers should use this drug with caution.

Relative infant dose:
Time to clear:
Lactation risk category: L4
Pregnancy risk category: C
Adult dose: 1 drop in the affected eye three times daily
Alternatives:

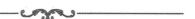

DOTHIEPIN

Trade names: Prothiaden, Dothep

AAP recommendation: Drug whose effect on nursing infants is unknown but may be of concern

Dothiepin is an antidepressant. It is transferred into breastmilk; however, no side effects were noted in breastfeeding infants. In an outcome study of 15 mother/infant pairs 3-5 years after birth, no behavior differences were noted in the dothiepin treated mothers/infants. This suggests that this drug did not change the cognitive abilities in the breastfed infants. In a study of 8 women, blood levels in 5 infants were very low. No side effects were noted in any of the infants following chronic maternal use.

Relative infant dose: 4.4%
Time to clear: Between 2.5 and 5 days
Lactation risk category: L2
Pregnancy risk category: D
Adult dose: 75-300 milligrams per day
Alternatives:

DOXAZOSIN MESYLATE

Trade names: Cardura, Carduran
AAP recommendation: Not reviewed

Doxazosin is used to treat hypertension (high blood pressure), among other uses. It is not known if doxazosin is transferred into breastmilk. Extreme caution is recommended.

Relative infant dose:
Time to clear: Between 1.5 and 4.5 days
Lactation risk category: L4
Pregnancy risk category: B
Adult dose: 2-4 milligrams daily
Alternatives: Propranolol, Metoprolol

DOXEPIN

Trade names: Adapin, Sinequan, Triadapin, Novo-Doxepin, Deptran
AAP recommendation: Drug whose effect on nursing infants is unknown but may be of concern

Doxepin is an antidepressant. Small but significant amounts are secreted in breastmilk. Two published reports showed that breastfeeding infants absorbed doxepin in amounts that varied from modest to significant. In one report, dangerous sedation and respiratory arrest was observed in a breastfeeding infant. Poor sucking and swallowing, muscle hypotonia, vomiting, drowsiness and jaudice in another breastfeeding infant have been reported, but these symptoms went after breastfeeding was stopped.

In another case report of a mother taking 35 milligrams per day, the infant was readmitted to the neonatal intensive care unit at the hospital on day 9 postpartum because of poor sucking and swallowing, muscle hypotonia, vomiting, drowsiness, and jaundice. This drug is not recommended for breastfeeding women.

Relative infant dose: 1.2%
Time to clear: Between 1.5 and 5 days
Lactation risk category: L5
Pregnancy risk category: C
Adult dose: 75-300 milligrams daily
Alternatives: Sertraline, Paroxetine

DOXEPIN CREAM

Trade names: Zonalon cream

AAP recommendation: Drug whose effect on nursing infants is unknown but may be of concern

Doxepin cream is an antihistamine-like cream used to treat severe itching. Small but significant amounts are secreted into breastmilk. See doxepin.

Relative infant dose:
Time to clear: Between 4.5 and 11 days
Lactation risk category: L4
Pregnancy risk category: B
Adult dose: 150-300 milligrams daily
Alternatives:

DOXYCYCLINE

Trade names: Doxychel, Vibramycin, Peristat, Doxycin, Vibra-Tabs, Doryx, Doxylin, Doxylar

AAP recommendation: Not reviewed

Doxycyline is an antibiotic and belongs to a class of antibiotics known as tetracyclines. Tetracyclines given orally to infants are known to discolor teeth and inhibit bone growth. Doxycycline and oxytetracycline stain teeth the least. Although most tetracyclines secreted into breastmilk are generally bound to calcium preventing their absorption, doxycycline is the least bound (20%) and may be better absorbed in a breastfeeding infant than other tetracyclines. Prolonged use could alter gastrointestinal flora and cause stained teeth. Short term use (less than 3 weeks) is probably okay. No harmful effects have been reported in breastfeeding infants, but prolonged use (months) is not advised.

Relative infant dose: 4.0%
Time to clear: Between 2.5 and 5 days
Lactation risk category: L3
L4 if used chronically
Pregnancy risk category: D
Adult dose: 100 milligrams daily
Alternatives:

DOXYLAMINE

Trade names: Unisom nighttime, Dozile, Mersyndol, Syndol, Panalgesic
AAP recommendation: Not reviewed

Doxylamine is an antihistamine with sedative properties. Doxylamine is a common ingredient in over-the-counter sleep aids. Like certain other sedating antihistamines, it should not be used in infants, particularly not in premature or newborn infants because it may either stimulate or sedate the infant. Levels in breastmilk are not known, but caution is recommended, particularly in infants with apnea or other respiratory syndromes.

Relative infant dose:
Time to clear: Between 40.4 and 50.5 hours
Lactation risk category: L4
Pregnancy risk category: B
Adult dose:
Alternatives:

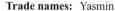

DROSPIRENONE

Trade names: Yasmin
AAP recommendation: Not reviewed

Drospirenone combined with ethinyl estradiol (30 micrograms) is marketed as the birth control product Yasmin. Drosperinone is poorly transferred into breastmilk. It contains estrogens (ethinyl estradiol) which are believed to strongly inhibit milk production in some women. Caution is recommended.

Relative infant dose:	1.3%
Time to clear:	Between 5 and 6.5 days
Lactation risk category:	L3
Pregnancy risk category:	X
Adult dose:	3 milligrams drosprenone per day
Alternatives:	Micronor

ECHINACEA

Trade names: Echinacea angustifolia, Echinacea purpurea, Antifect, Snakeroot, American Cone Flower, Black Susans

AAP recommendation: Not reviewed

Echinacea is a popular herbal remedy. It has traditionally been used on the skin to stimulate wound healing and internally to stimulate the immune system. The plant contains a complex mixture of compounds and no single compound appears to be responsible for its immuno-stimulant properties. To date, little is known about the toxicity of this plant; although, its use has been widespread for many years. Echinacea should not be used in patients with autoimmune syndromes such as multiple sclerosis, diabetes mellitus, etc. It appears that purified Echinacea extract is relatively non-toxic even at high doses. There are no reports on its transfer into breastmilk or its effect on lactation. It should probably not be used for more than 8 weeks. As with all herbals, their potential for risk should always be considered in young breastfeeding infants.

Relative infant dose:	
Time to clear:	
Lactation risk category:	L3
Pregnancy risk category:	
Adult dose:	
Alternatives:	

ELETRIPTAN

Trade names: Relpax

AAP recommendation: Not reviewed

Eletriptan is used to treat migraine headaches. Eletriptan is poorly transferred into breastmilk. The manufacturer reports that in one study of 8 women given a single dose of 80 milligrams eletriptan, the average amount of eletriptan in breastmilk over 24 hours was approximately 0.02%. It is not likely that the dose the breastfeeding infant would receive would be harmful.

Relative infant dose:	0.02%
Time to clear:	Between 16 and 20 hours
Lactation risk category:	L2
Pregnancy risk category:	C
Adult dose:	20-40 milligrams initially for headache. One repeat dose after 2 hours if needed.
Alternatives:	Sumatriptan

ENALAPRIL MALEATE

Trade names: Vasotec, Amprace, Renitec, Innovace

AAP recommendation: Maternal medication usually compatible with breastfeeding

Enalapril maleate is used to treat hypertension (high blood pressure). In two studies, the amount of enalapril transferred into breastmilk was low. Until there is more information on drug transfer into breastmilk, this drug should be used with caution in breastfeeding women, especially right after birth.

Relative infant dose:	0.2%
Time to clear:	Between 6 and 7 days
Lactation risk category:	L2
Pregnancy risk category:	C if used during 1st trimester
	D if used during 2nd and 3rd trimesters
Adult dose:	10-40 milligrams daily
Alternatives:	Captopril, Benazepril

ENOXACIN

Trade names: Penetrex, Enoxin, Comprecin

AAP recommendation: Not reviewed

Enoxacin is an antibiotic similar to ciprofloxacin (Cipro). There are no reports on the transfer of enoxacin into breastmilk. See ofloxacin and norfloxacin as alternatives. Changes in gut flora and diarrhea could occur in breastfed infants.

Relative infant dose:
Time to clear: Between 12 and 30 hours
Lactation risk category: L3
Pregnancy risk category: C
Adult dose: 200-400 milligrams twice daily
Alternatives: Ofloxacin, Norfloxacin, Ciprofloxacin

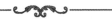

EPSTEIN-BARR VIRUS

Common names: Mononucleosis, EBV

AAP recommendation: Not reviewed

The Epstein-Barr virus (EBV) is the cause of infectious mononucleosis, a disease that causes swollen lymph nodes, fever, and a high white blood cell count. It is not known if EBV is secreted into breastmilk; although, it is likely. Breastmilk is not believed to be a significant source of early EBV infections so mothers with EBV may breastfeed.

Relative infant dose:
Time to clear:
Lactation risk category: L3
Pregnancy risk category:
Adult dose:
Alternatives:

ERGONOVINE MALEATE

Trade names: Ergotrate, Ergometrine, Syntometrine

AAP recommendation: Not reviewed

Ergonovine is used to prevent and treat postpartum hemorrhage (bleeding), among other uses. Ergonovine use in lactating women would probably suppress lactation. Although ergonovine is transferred into breastmilk, one study proposed that use of ergonovine during breastfeeding would not affect the infant. When used at doses of 0.2 milligrams up to 3-4 times daily, only small quantities of ergonovine was found in the breastmilk. Methylergonovine is preferred because it produces less hypertension (high blood pressure) than ergonovine, does not inhibit lactation, and the levels in breastmilk are minimal. See monograph for methylergovonine.

Short-term (1 week) low-dose regimens of these drugs do not appear to pose problems in nursing mothers or their infants, but it is risky. Methylergonovine is preferred because it does not inhibit lactation and levels in milk are minimal. However, the prolonged use (weeks) of ergot alkaloids should be avoided and could possibly lead to severe gangrene.

Relative infant dose: 2.2%
Time to clear: Between 2 and 10 hours
Lactation risk category: L3
Pregnancy risk category: X
Adult dose: 0.2 milligrams injected into the muscle every 2-4 hours
Alternatives: Methylergonovine

ERGOTAMINE TARTRATE

Trade names: Wigraine, Cafergot, Ergostat, Ergomar,
DHE-45, Gynergen, Ergodryl, Migral, Lingraine

AAP recommendation: Drug associated with significant side effects and
should be taken with caution

Ergotamine is used to treat the acute phase of a migraine headache. Although early reports suggest ergotamine compounds are secreted into breastmilk and cause vomiting and diarrhea in infants, other authors suggest that the short term use of ergotamine (0.2 milligram postpartum) generally presents no problem to a nursing infant. This is likely because less than 5% of ergotamine is orally absorbed in adults. Excessive dosing and long-term use may suppress milk production. Use during lactation is strongly discouraged.

Relative infant dose:
Time to clear: Between 3.5 and 4.5 days
Lactation risk category: L4
Pregnancy risk category: X
Adult dose: 2 milligrams every 30 minutes
Alternatives: Propranolol, Sumatriptan

ERYTHROMYCIN

Trade names: E-Mycin, ERY-TAB, ERYC, Ilosone, Eryc,
Erythromide, Novo-Rythro, PCE, Ilotyc, EMU-V, EES,
Erythrocin, Ceplac, Erycen

AAP recommendation: Maternal medication usually compatible with
breastfeeding

Erythromycin is an antibiotic. There is strong evidence that the use of erythromycin in breastfeeding mothers causes pyloric stenosis in infants. Pyloric stenosis is the abnormal enlargement of the muscles of the pylorus (the opening between the stomach and duodenum). This usually occurs in infants 3-10 weeks of age. See azithromycin as an alternative.

Relative infant dose: 1.7%
Time to clear: Between 6 and 10 hours
Lactation risk category: L1
    L3 early postnatally (pyloric stenosis)
Pregnancy risk category: B
Adult dose: 500-800 milligrams four times daily
Alternatives: Azithromycin, Clarithromycin

ESCITALOPRAM

Trade names: Lexapro
AAP recommendation: Not reviewed

Escitalpram is used to treat depression. Escitalopram is the active metabolite of citalopram. Two cases of sleepiness in breastfeeding infants have been reported by the manufacturer following the use of citalopram. This author has had numerous reports of sleepy infants (generally newborns) after the use of Escitalpram as well. There are no reports on the transfer of escitalopram into breastmilk. Because this drug is identical to citalopram, the transfer into breastmilk should be the same. See citalopram. Until we know more about the effect of escitalopram on breastfeeding infants, great caution is recommended, particularly with newborns. Observe infant for sleepiness.

Relative infant dose:
Time to clear: Between 4.5 and 6.5 days
Lactation risk category: L3 in older infants
Pregnancy risk category: C
Adult dose: 10-40 milligrams daily
Alternatives: Sertraline, Paroxetine, Bupropion, Venlafaxine

ESOMEPRAZOLE

Trade names: Nexium
AAP recommendation: Not reviewed

Esomeprazole is closely related to omeprazole. See omeprazole for breastfeeding recommendations.

Relative infant dose:
Time to clear:
Lactation risk category:　　L2
Pregnancy risk category:　　C
Adult dose:
Alternatives:

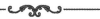

ESTROGEN-ESTRADIOL

Trade names:　Estratab, Premarin, Menest, Estraderm,
　　　　　　　　　Delestrogen, Estinyl, Estring, Evorel

AAP recommendation:　Maternal medication usually compatible with
　　　　　　　　　　　　breastfeeding

Estrogen is a hormone. Although small amounts may pass into breastmilk, it appears to have very little effect on the infant. The use of estrogens early postpartum may reduce the volume of milk produced and the protein content in the milk. This varies and depends on the individual and the dose taken. Breastfeeding mothers should wait until lactation is firmly established (6-8 weeks) before starting estrogen-containing oral contraceptives. If oral contraceptives are used during lactation, the transfer of estradiol into breastmilk will be low and does not exceed the amount normally transferred when the mother resumes ovulation. However, progesin-only birth control pills are greatly preferred in breastfeeding mothers. See oral contraceptives.

Relative infant dose:
Time to clear:　　　　　　　Between 4 and 5 hours
Lactation risk category:　　L3
Pregnancy risk category:　　X
Adult dose:　　10 milligrams three times daily
Alternatives:　Norethindrone

ETHANOL

Common names:　Alcohol

AAP recommendation:　Maternal medication usually compatible with
　　　　　　　　　　　　breastfeeding

The alcohol found in beer, wines, and other drinks is more correctly called ethanol. The amount of alcohol transferred into breastmilk is the same as the amount in the mother's blood. When use infrequently and with a brief waiting period, the small amounts present in milk do not seem to be harmful to the infant, although each infant should be evaluated separately (premature infants may be exceedingly sensitive; do not use alcohol if you have a premature infant).

Beer, but not other forms of alcohol, has been reported in a number of studies to increase prolactin levels and breastmilk production. It is presumed that the polysaccharide from barley may be the prolactin-stimulating component of beer. Non-alcoholic beer is equally effective. A study that was performed with alcohol mixed with orange juice caused an increase in breastmilk odor. Excess alcohol blood levels may lead to drowsiness, deep sleep, weakness, and decreased linear growth in breastfeeding infants. Other studies have suggested psychomotor delay in infants of moderate drinkers (2+ drinks daily).

Avoid breastfeeding during and 2-3 hours after drinking alcohol. In an interesting study of the effect of alcohol on milk ingestion by infants, infants consumed significantly less milk during the 4 hours immediately after exposure to alcohol. Eight to sixteen hours after exposure, the infants increased their milk intake if their mothers refrained from drinking. Some infants may not like the taste of alcohol in milk which may account for the reduced consumption during this interval. Adults break down 1 ounce of alcohol in about 3 hours.

Mothers who ingest alcohol in moderate amounts can generally return to breastfeeding as soon as they no longer feel the effects of the alcohol. The best advice is to wait one hour for each drink ingested. Thus if you drink two glasses of wine, wait at least 2 hours or more before breastfeeding. Chronic or heavy consumers of alcohol should not breastfeed.

Relative infant dose:	16%
Time to clear:	Between 57.5 and 72 minutes
Lactation risk category:	L3
Pregnancy risk category:	D
Adult dose:	
Alternatives:	

ETHOSUXIMIDE

Trade names: Zarontin

AAP recommendation: Maternal medication usually compatible with breastfeeding

Ethosuximide is an anticonvulsant used in epilepsy. Significant amounts of ethosuximide are transferred into breastmilk, but blood levels of ethosuximide in breastfeeding infants are considered to be too low to produce an effect. It is suggested that the infant's blood levels be occasionally tested if the mother takes ethosuximide. The infant may have a poor suck, be sleepy, and/or be very excitable. Caution is recommended.

Relative infant dose: 31.5%
Time to clear: Between 5 and 12.5 days
Lactation risk category: L4
Pregnancy risk category: C
Adult dose: 250-750 milligrams twice daily
Alternatives:

ETIDRONATE

Trade names: Didronel

AAP recommendation: Not reviewed

Etidronate is used to treat the symptoms of a particular bone-softening syndrome (Paget's). There are no reports on the transfer of etidronate into breastmilk; although, it might be possible. It is not known if etidronate affects the breastfeeding infant's bones. However, due to the presence of fat and calcium in milk, the oral absorption of etidronate in infants would be exceedingly low. It is possible that the drug could reduce the levels of calcium in breastmilk, but this has not been reported.

Relative infant dose:
Time to clear: Between 24 and 30 hours
Lactation risk category: L3
Pregnancy risk category: B
Adult dose: 5-10 milligrams per kilogram per day
Alternatives:

ETONOGESTREL AND ETHINYL ESTRADIOL

Trade names: NuvaRing

AAP recommendation: Not reviewed

NuvaRing is a slow release vaginal ring which releases etonogestrel and ethinyl estradiol over a 3 week period. The amount of ethinyl estradiol absorbed into the blood is about the same whether the drug is inserted into the vagina or taken by mouth. Small amounts of estrogens and progestins are known to pass into milk, but long-term follow-up of children whose mothers used combination hormonal contraceptives while breastfeeding has shown no harmful effects in infants. Estrogen-containing contraceptives may interfere with milk production by decreasing the quantity and quality of breastmilk. Some caution is recommended due to its estrogen content.

Relative infant dose:
Time to clear: Between 5 and 6 days
Lactation risk category: L3
Pregnancy risk category: X
Adult dose:
Alternatives: Progestin-only oral contraceptives.

ETONOGESTREL IMPLANT

Trade names: Implanon

AAP recommendation: Not reviewed

Implanon (etonogestrel) is a non-biodegradable contraceptive single-rod implant which releases etonogestrel over a 3 year period. Small amounts of progestins are known to pass into milk. However, long-term follow-up of children whose mothers used hormonal contraceptives while breastfeeding has shown no harmful effects on infants. Of the contraceptives, progestins are generally preferred as they produce fewer changes in milk production compared to estrogen-containing products. This product is probably quite safe for use in breastfeeding mothers, but mothers should watch for changes in milk production. Some mothers (rare) appear quite sensitive to progestins and should not use while breastfeeding.

Relative infant dose:
Time to clear: Between 5 and 6 days
Lactation risk category: L2
Pregnancy risk category: X
Adult dose: One implant every 3 years
Alternatives: Norethindrone

EVENING PRIMROSE OIL

Common names: EPO

AAP recommendation: Not reviewed

Evening primrose oil has a wide spectrum of uses. It is a rich source of essential polyunsaturated fatty acids (EFA), particularly gamma linoleic acid

(GLA). Women who take EFA during pregnancy have much higher levels of EFA in their breastmilk. Toxicity of this product appears quite low.

Relative infant dose:
Time to clear:
Lactation risk category: L3
Pregnancy risk category:
Adult dose:
Alternatives:

FAMCICLOVIR

Trade names: Famvir
AAP recommendation: Not reviewed

Famciclovir is an antiviral agent used to treat herpes zoster infection (shingles) and genital herpes. Although similar to acyclovir, there are no reports on the levels of famciclovir in breastmilk. Since famciclovir provides few advantages over acyclovir, acyclovir is preferred in nursing mothers.

Relative infant dose:
Time to clear: Between 8 and 15 hours
Lactation risk category: L2
Pregnancy risk category: B
Adult dose: 125 milligrams twice daily
Alternatives: Acyclovir

FAMOTIDINE

Trade names: Pepcid, Axid-AR, Pepcid-AC, Amfamox, Apo-Famotidine, Pepcidine, Novo-Famotidine
AAP recommendation: Not reviewed

Famotidine is used to treat duodenal and gastric ulcers, stomach acidity, and other uses. Famotidine is transferred into breastmilk, but levels seem to be much lower than the levels of other drugs in the same class (e.g. ranitidine, cimetidine). Famotidine is, therefore, the preferred drug.

Relative infant dose: 1.9%
Time to clear: Between 10 and 17.5 hours
Lactation risk category: L1
Pregnancy risk category: B

Adult dose: 20-40 milligrams twice daily
Alternatives: Nizatidine

FELODIPINE

Trade names: Plendil, Renedil, Agon SR, Plendil ER
AAP recommendation: Not reviewed

Felodipine is used to treat hypertension (high blood pressure). Because we have numerous studies on other drugs in this family, it is advisable to use nifedipine or others that have been studied in breastfeeding mothers.

Relative infant dose:
Time to clear: Between 2 and 3.5 days
Lactation risk category: L3
Pregnancy risk category: C
Adult dose: 2.5-10 milligrams daily
Alternatives: Nifedipine, Nimodipine, Verapamil

FENNEL

Common names: Sweet Fennel, Bitter fennel, Carosella,
                   Florence fennel, Finocchio, Garden fennel, Wild fennel
AAP recommendation: Not reviewed

Fennel is an ancient herb native to southern Europe and Asia. It is reputed to increase milk secretion, promote menstruation, facilitate birth, and increase libido. Ingestion of the volatile oil may cause nausea, vomiting, seizures, pulmonary edema and hallucinations. It is believed to be estrogenic. Because estrogens are known to suppress breastmilk production, its use in breastfeeding women is questionable.

Relative infant dose:
Time to clear:
Lactation risk category: L4
Pregnancy risk category:
Adult dose:
Alternatives:

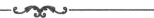

FENOPROFEN

Trade names: Nalfon, Fenopron, Progesic

AAP recommendation: Not reviewed

Fenoprofen is used to treat rheumatoid arthritis, osteoarthritis, and to relieve mild to moderate pain. Trace amounts of fenoprofen transfer into breastmilk. Fenoprofen was undetectable in cord blood, amniotic fluid, saliva, or washed red blood cells after multiple doses.

Relative infant dose:
Time to clear: Between 10 and 12.5 hours
Lactation risk category: L2
Pregnancy risk category: B during 1st and 2nd trimesters
D during 3rd trimester
Adult dose: 300-600 milligrams every 4-6 hours
Alternatives: Ibuprofen

FENTANYL

Trade names: Sublimaze, Duragesic

AAP recommendation: Maternal medication usually compatible with breastfeeding

Fentanyl is a potent narcotic pain killer used (IV, IM, topically) during labor and delivery, and in other painful syndromes. When used by injection, its half-life is very short. The transfer of fentanyl into breastmilk has been studied and is reportedly very low. In two studies, the amount of fentanyl in milk was very low, sometimes even undetectable. Since there are small amounts in milk and it is poorly absorbed when taken by mouth, it is unlikely to have a harmful effect on a breastfeeding infant.

Relative infant dose: 3%
Time to clear: Between 8 and 20 hours
Lactation risk category: L2
Pregnancy risk category: B
Adult dose: 2-20 micrograms per kilogram intravenous injection
Alternatives:

FENUGREEK

Trade names:

AAP recommendation: Not reviewed

Fenugreek is commonly sold as a dried, ripe seed. Extracts of fenugreek are used as an artificial flavor for maple syrup. The transfer of fenugreek into breastmilk is unknown, but harmful effects have only rarely been reported. One case of gastrointestinal bleeding in a premature infant (30 weeks) after the mother began taking fenugreek has been reported.

It has been speculated that fenugreek caused the bleeding, but this has not been proven. In a group of 10 women who took 3 fenugreek capsules 3 times daily (Nature's Way) for a week, the average milk production during the week more than doubled (mean of 207 milliliters per day to 464 milliliters per day). No harmful effects were reported. When taken in moderation, fenugreek has limited toxicity. A maple syrup odor in the urine and sweat is commonly reported in the infant. Higher doses may produce hypoglycemia (low blood sugar levels). Its use in late pregnancy may not be advisable.

Relative infant dose:
Time to clear:
Lactation risk category: L3
Pregnancy risk category:
Adult dose:
Alternatives: Metoclopramide, Domperidone

FEXOFENADINE

Trade names: Allegra

AAP recommendation: Maternal medication usually compatible with breastfeeding

Fexofenadine is a non-sedating antihistamine used to treat nasal and other allergies. In a study in which women received terfenadine, only small amounts of fexofenadine were found in breastmilk. The authors estimate that only 0.45% of the maternal dose would be ingested by the infant.

Relative infant dose: 0.7%
Time to clear: Between 2.5 and 3 days
Lactation risk category: L2
Pregnancy risk category: C
Adult dose: 60 milligrams twice daily

Alternatives:

FLAVOXATE

Trade names: Urispas
AAP recommendation: Not reviewed

Flavoxate is used as an antispasmodic to provide relief of painful urination, urgency, nocturia (excessive urination at night), urinary frequency or incontinence. There are no reports on the transfer of flavoxate into breastmilk.

Relative infant dose:
Time to clear: Between 40 and 50 hours
Lactation risk category: L3
Pregnancy risk category: B
Adult dose: 100-200 milligrams three to four times daily
Alternatives:

FLOXACILLIN

Trade names: Flucil, Flucloxacillin, Flopen, Floxapen,
                Staphylex, Flu-Amp, Flu-Clomix, Magnapen
AAP recommendation: Not reviewed

Floxacillin, also called flucloxacillin, is a penicillin antibiotic. Only trace amounts of floxacillin are secreted into breastmilk. A similar drug, cloxacillin, is commonly used to treat mastitis (infection of the breasts) in breastfeeding mothers and has been used in thousands of breastfeeding patients without a problem. Changes in gut flora are possible but unlikely.

Relative infant dose:
Time to clear: Between 6 and 7.5 hours
Lactation risk category: L1
Pregnancy risk category: B
Adult dose: 250-500 milligrams four times daily
Alternatives: Cloxacillin, Dicloxacillin

FLUCONAZOLE

Trade names: Diflucan

AAP recommendation: Maternal medication usually compatible with breastfeeding

Fluconazole is an antifungal agent that is frequently used for vaginal, oral and esophageal candida infections. Oral fluconazole is currently cleared for pediatric candidiasis for infants 6 months and older and has an FDA Safety Profile for neonates 1 day and older. Moderate amounts of fluconazole (< 16%) transfer to the infant via milk. This is far less than the clinical dose given to an infant to treat infections. This drug is considered relatively safe for breastfeeding mothers.

Relative infant dose: 16.1%
Time to clear: Between 5 and 6.5 days
Lactation risk category: L2
Pregnancy risk category: C
Adult dose: 50-200 milligrams daily
Alternatives:

FLUNARIZINE

Trade names: Sibelium, Novo-Flunarizine

AAP recommendation: Not reviewed

Flunarizine is used to treat hypertension (high blood pressure) and migraine headaches. There are no reports on the transfer of flunarizine into breastmilk. However, it is possible that flunarizine can build up over time and concentrate in a breastfed infant. Other drugs in the same class as flunarizine may be preferred. Use with extreme caution.

Relative infant dose:
Time to clear: Between 76 and 95 days
Lactation risk category: L4
Pregnancy risk category:
Adult dose: 10 milligrams daily
Alternatives: Nifedipine, Nimodipine, Verapamil

FLUNISOLIDE

Trade names: Nasalide, Aerobid, Rhinalar, Syntaris, PMS-Flunisolide

AAP recommendation: Not reviewed

Flunisolide is a potent steroid used to treat symptoms in asthmatics. It is also available in Nasalide for intranasal use for allergic rhinitis (nasal allergies). Generally, only small levels of flunisolide are absorbed (about 40%) and milk levels would likely be low. Although there are no reports on breastmilk levels, it is unlikely that the level secreted in milk is clinically relevant.

Relative infant dose:
Time to clear: Between 7 and 9 hours
Lactation risk category: L3
Pregnancy risk category: C
Adult dose: 1 milligram daily
Alternatives:

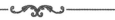

FLUNITRAZEPAM

Trade names: Rohypnol, Hypnodorm, Raohypnol

AAP recommendation: Not reviewed

Flunitrazepam is frequently called the "Date Rape Pill". Flunitrazepam induces rapid sleep and loss of short term memory, particularly when mixed with alcohol. The effects last about 8 hours. It is recommended to induce adult insomnia and for pediatric preanesthetic sedation. Flunitrazepam is not available in the USA and is probably not appropriate for breastfeeding mothers.

Relative infant dose:
Time to clear: Between 3.5 and 6.5 days
Lactation risk category: L3
L4 if used chronically
Pregnancy risk category: D
Adult dose: 2 milligrams daily
Alternatives: Lorazepam, Alprazolam

FLUORIDE

Trade names: Pediaflor, Flura, Fluotic, Fluor-A-Day, Fluorigard

AAP recommendation: Reported as having no effect on breastfeeding

Fluoride is an essential element required for bone and teeth development. Excessive levels are known to permanently stain teeth. Fluoride likely forms calcium fluoride salts in milk which may limit the amount of fluoride absorbed from breastmilk. Mothers do not need fluoride supplements if the water in their area has more than 0.7 ppm. One infant has been reported to be allergic to fluoride. Younger children (2-6 yrs) should use a very small amount of toothpaste and not to swallow it. The American Academy of Pediatrics (AAP) no longer recommends giving breastfed infants oral fluoride.

Relative infant dose:
Time to clear: Between 24 and 30 hours
Lactation risk category: L2
Pregnancy risk category: C
Adult dose: 1 milligram daily
Alternatives:

FLUOXETINE

Trade names: Prozac, Serafem, Apo-Fluoxetine, Lovan, Novo-Fluoxetine, Zactin

AAP recommendation: Drug whose effect on nursing infants is unknown but may be of concern

Fluoxetine is a very popular antidepressant that is also used for a host of other syndromes. Fluoxetine is rapidly and completely absorbed. At present, fluoxetine is the only antidepressant cleared for use in pregnancy. This may pose an added problem in breastfed infants. Infants born of mothers receiving fluoxetine have fluoxetine in their system. Each time they are breastfed their level of fluoxetine may increase.

Four case reports of side effects have been published and include side effects such as coma, sleepiness, seizures, colic, fussiness, and prolonged crying. Methods to reduce exposure of the breastfed infant include: reduce the dose several weeks prior to delivery (or even after delivery), switch to a safer antidepressant prior to or after delivery. If the patient cannot tolerate switching to another antidepressant, then fluoxetine and breastfeeding should be continued.

The age of the infant when fluoxetine therapy is started is important. Use in older infants (4-6 months or older) is far less harmful because they can break down and get rid of the medication easily. Current reports on Sertraline and Paroxetine suggest that these medications have difficulty entering milk, and more importantly, the infant. Therefore, they are preferred over fluoxetine for therapy of depression in breastfeeding mothers.

However, it is important to remember that the risks of not breastfeeding far outweigh the risk of using fluoxetine. Women who can only take fluoxetine should continue breastfeeding and observe the infant for side effects.

Relative infant dose:	6.8%
Time to clear:	Between 8 and 15 days
Lactation risk category:	L2 in older infants
	L3 if used in neonatal period
Pregnancy risk category:	B
Adult dose:	20-40 milligrams daily
Alternatives:	Sertraline, Paroxetine, Citalopram

FLUPHENAZINE

Trade names: Prolixin, Permitil, Modecate, Moditen, Anatensol

AAP recommendation: Not reviewed

Fluphenazine is a potent tranquilizer used to treat psychotic disorders and schizophrenia. There are no reports on the transfer of fluphenazine into breastmilk.

Relative infant dose:	
Time to clear:	Between 1.5 and 4 days
Lactation risk category:	L3
Pregnancy risk category:	C
Adult dose:	1-5 milligrams daily
Alternatives:	

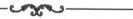

FLURAZEPAM

Trade names: Dalmane, Novo-Flupam

AAP recommendation: Not reviewed

Flurazepam is a sedative generally used to treat insomnia (sleeplessness). Because most drugs in the same class as flurazepam are secreted into breastmilk, flurazepam entry into milk should be expected. However, there are no specific reports on the levels of flurazepam in breastmilk. See diazepam.

Relative infant dose:
Time to clear: Between 8 and 21 days
Lactation risk category: L3
Pregnancy risk category: X
Adult dose: 15-30 milligrams daily
Alternatives: Lorazepam, Alprazolam

FLURBIPROFEN

Trade names: Ansaid, Froben, Ocufen
AAP recommendation: Not reviewed

Flurbiprofen is a pain killer similar to ibuprofen. It is used both as an ophthalmic (eye) preparation and orally (by mouth). In a study of 12 women, the amount of flurbiprofen in milk was very low. Amounts in breastmilk and plasma of nursing mothers suggest that a nursing infant would receive less than 0.1 milligrams flurbiprofen per day, a level considered very low. These studies suggest that the amount of flurbiprofen transferred into breastmilk would not be harmful to the infant.

Relative infant dose:
Time to clear: Between 15 and 28.5 hours
Lactation risk category: L2
Pregnancy risk category: B during 1st and 2nd trimester
C during 3rd trimester
Adult dose: 200-300 milligrams daily
Alternatives: Ibuprofen

FLUTICASONE

Trade names: Flonase, Flovent, Cutivate, Flixotide, Flixonase
AAP recommendation: Not reviewed

Fluticasone is used intranasally for allergies and is also available in inhalers for asthma. When fluticasone is used intranasally, almost no drug is absorbed into the blood. When fluticasone is taken orally, most of the drug is broken down by the liver. Therefore, due to its poor absorption, little or no drug is likely present in milk.

Relative infant dose:
Time to clear: Between 31 and 39 hours
Lactation risk category: L3
Pregnancy risk category: C
Adult dose: 50-110 micrograms daily per inhalation
Alternatives:

FLUTICASONE AND SALMETEROL

Trade names: Advair

AAP recommendation: Not reviewed

Advair combines fluticasone and salmeterol and is used to treat asthma. See fluticasone (Flovent) and salmeterol (Serevent). Due to the poor absorption of these two drugs, little or none is likely to enter milk.

Relative infant dose:
Time to clear:
Lactation risk category: L3
Pregnancy risk category:
Adult dose:
Alternatives:

FLUVOXAMINE

Trade names: Luvox, Apo-Fluvoxamine, Alti-Fluvoxamine, Faverin, Floxyfral, Myroxim

AAP recommendation: Drug whose effect on nursing infants is unknown but may be of concern

Fluvoxamine is mainly used to treat obsessive-compulsive disorders (OCD). Only very small amounts of fluvoxamine are transferred to infants (< 1.5%). No harmful effects have been noted and infants show normal development. According to the authors in one study, the infants suffered no side effects as a result of this intake and this drug poses little risk to a nursing infant. In summary, the data from the 8 studies suggests that only very small amounts of fluvoxamine are transferred to infants, that plasma levels in infants are too low to be detected, and no harmful effects have been noted.

Relative infant dose: 1.4%
Time to clear: Between 2.5 and 3 days

Lactation risk category: L2
Pregnancy risk category: C
Adult dose: 50-300 milligrams daily
Alternatives: Sertraline, Paroxetine

FOLIC ACID

Trade names: Folacin, Wellcovorin, Folvite, Novo-Folacid, Accomin, Bioglan Daily, Megafol

AAP recommendation: Maternal medication usually compatible with breastfeeding

Folic acid is an essential vitamin. Individuals most likely to be low in folic acid are pregnant patients and those receiving anticonvulsants or birth control pills. Infant spinal cord problems have been shown to be reduced when their mothers took additional folic acid. Women are strongly urged to take folic acid prior to and during pregnancy. Folic acid is actively secreted into breastmilk, even if levels in the mother are low. High doses (greater than 1 milligram per day) should not be taken by pregnant and breastfeeding women. The infant receives the right amount of folic acid from a normal milk supply.

Relative infant dose: 47.8%
Time to clear:
Lactation risk category: L1
Pregnancy risk category: A during 1st and 2nd trimester
C during 3rd trimester
Adult dose: 0.4-0.8 milligrams daily
Alternatives:

FOSINOPRIL

Trade names: Monopril, Staril

AAP recommendation: Not reviewed

Fosinopril is broken down to fosinoprilat by the liver. Fosinoprilat is used to lower high blood pressure. The manufacturer reports that taking 20 milligrams daily for three days resulted in barely detectable levels in breastmilk, although no values were provided. See enalapril, benazepril, captopril as alternatives.

Relative infant dose:

Time to clear: Between 2 and 7.5 days
Lactation risk category: L3
                               L4 if used in premature infants
Pregnancy risk category: D
Adult dose: 20-40 milligrams daily
Alternatives: Enalapril, Benazepril, Captopril

FOSPHENYTOIN

Trade names: Cerebyx

AAP recommendation: Maternal medication usually compatible with
                        breastfeeding

Fosphenytoin is broken down to form phenytoin, an anticonvulsant. See
phenytoin for breastmilk specifics.

Relative infant dose:
Time to clear: Between 60 and 75 minutes
Lactation risk category: L2
Pregnancy risk category: D
Adult dose: 4-6 milligrams phenytoin equivalents per kilogram per day
Alternatives: Phenytoin

FROVATRIPTAN SUCCINATE

Trade names: Frova

AAP recommendation: Not reviewed

Frovatriptan is used to treat migraine headaches. There are no reports on the
transfer of frovatriptan into breastmilk. The authors recommend sumatriptan
as an alternative. Good data suggests that milk levels of sumatriptan are low
and its oral absorption is low.

Relative infant dose:
Time to clear: Between 4.5 and 5.5 days
Lactation risk category: L3
Pregnancy risk category: C
Adult dose: 2.5 milligrams initially followed by one dose after 2 hours
                  if no response.
Alternatives: Sumatriptan

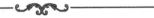

FURAZOLIDONE

Trade names: Furoxone

AAP recommendation: Not reviewed

Furazolidone belongs to the nitrofurantoin family of antibiotics (see nitrofurantoin). Following an oral dose, furazolidone was poorly absorbed (less than 5%). It is largely inactivated in the gut. Amounts transferred into breastmilk are unreported, but the total amounts would be very low due to the low amounts in the maternal blood. The breastfeeding infant would be unlikely to absorb very much of this drug from breastmilk. Caution should be observed in early postpartum newborns due to the effect of this drug on bilirubin.

Relative infant dose:
Time to clear:
Lactation risk category: L2
                                    L4 early postpartum
Pregnancy risk category: C
Adult dose: 100 milligrams four times daily
Alternatives:

FUROSEMIDE

Trade names: Lasix, Novo-Semide, Frusemide, Uremide,
                   Frusid

AAP recommendation: Not reviewed

Furosemide is a diuretic that increases the flow of urine. It has been found in breastmilk, but the levels are unreported. Diuretics, by reducing blood volume, could reduce breastmilk supply; although, this is largely theory and has not been proven. Furosemide is often used in newborns in pediatric units. Very little is absorbed by newborns and very high oral doses are required in infants. It is very unlikely that the amount of furosemide transferred into breastmilk would produce any effects in a nursing infant.

Relative infant dose:
Time to clear: Between 6 and 7.5 hours
Lactation risk category: L3
Pregnancy risk category: C
Adult dose: 40-80 milligrams twice daily
Alternatives:

GABAPENTIN

Trade names: Neurontin

AAP recommendation: Not reviewed

Gabapentin is a newer anticonvulsant used mainly to treat seizures. There are no reports on the transfer of gabapentin into breastmilk. However, in preliminary results from a study of two breastfeeding mothers who received gabapentin in my laboratories, no harmful effects were noted in the infants.

Relative infant dose:	6.6%
Time to clear:	Between 20 and 35 hours
Lactation risk category:	L3
Pregnancy risk category:	C
Adult dose:	300-600 milligrams three times daily
Alternatives:	

GATIFLOXACIN

Trade names: Tequin, Zymar

AAP recommendation: Not reviewed

Gatifloxacin is a member of the fluoroquinolone antibiotic family. It is similar to ofloxacin, levofloxacin, and ciprofloxacin. Its use in pediatric patients is not generally recommended; although, newer reports suggest that this family is safe in pediatric patients. There are no reports on the transfer of gatifloxacin into breastmilk. Of the many fluoroquinolone antibiotics, ofloxacin and levofloxacin are probably preferred in breastfeeding patients due to lower milk levels. The only major risk to an infant is a change in gut flora and a gut infection due to overgrowth of dangerous bacteria. If used, observe infant for bloody diarrhea. Ophthalmic Product (Gatifloxacin): There are no reports on its transfer into human milk. Ophthalmic (eye solution) exposure is very unlikely to produce harmful levels in breastmilk. The fluoroquinolones are becoming more popular for use in pediatric patients due to a number of recent studies and reviews.

Relative infant dose:	
Time to clear:	Between 28.5 and 35.5 hours
Lactation risk category:	L3
Pregnancy risk category:	C
Adult dose:	400 milligrams daily
Alternatives:	Ofloxacin, Levofloxacin

GENTAMICIN

Trade names: Garamycin, Cidomycin, Garatec, Palacos, Septopal

AAP recommendation: Not reviewed

Gentamicin is an antibiotic. When taken orally, the amount absorbed is less than 1%. Premature babies are an exception - they may absorb small amounts. In one study, it was found that blood levels of gentamicin in newborns were small and were found in only 5 of the 10 babies. The authors estimate that the daily amount of gentamicin from breastmilk would not be harmful in most infants. Gentamicin is commonly use in premature infants in our neonatal intensive care units.

Relative infant dose:	2.1%
Time to clear:	Between 8 and 15 hours
Lactation risk category:	L2
Pregnancy risk category:	C
Adult dose:	1.5-2.5 milligrams per kilogram every 8 hours
Alternatives:	

GENTIAN VIOLET

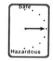

Trade names: Crystal violet, Methylrosailine chloride, Gentian Violet

AAP recommendation: Not reviewed

Gentian violet is an older product that, when used on the skin and in the mouth is a very effective antifungal and antimicrobial. It is a strong purple dye that is difficult to remove. Gentian violet has been found to have the same effect as other antifungals and is much better than nystatin in treating oral (not esophageal) candida (yeast) infections in patients with advanced AIDS.

Gentian violet solutions generally come as 1-2% gentian violet dissolved in a 10% solution of alcohol. For use with infants, the solution should be diluted with distilled water to 0.25 to 0.5% gentian violet. This makes gentian violet less likely to irritate the skin and reduces the alcohol content. When applied to the nipple, the alcohol may irritate the nipple, but it is not harmful to the infant. Gentian violet, when used in higher concentrations (> 1%), or for more than 7 days, is known to be very irritating, leading to ulcers in the mouth of children. Long-term use will lead to severe irritation of the infant's mouth. To use, soak a small swab in the solution, then have the baby suck on the swab or apply it directly to the affected areas in the mouth no more than once or twice daily for no more than 3-7 days. If the mother has Candidiasis on her nipple, Gentian Violet can be applied to the nipple area. Remember, do not use more than 7 days.

Relative infant dose:
Time to clear:
Lactation risk category: L3
Pregnancy risk category: C
Adult dose:
Alternatives:

GINKGO BILOBA

Common names: Ginko

AAP recommendation: Not reviewed

Ginkgo Biloba (GBE) is the world's oldest living tree. Extracts of the leaves contain many helpful compounds. The seeds contain ginkgo toxin, which is particularly toxic, and should not be consumed. Many studies reviewing ginkgo have been reported. It is used to treat cerebral insufficiency, asthma, dementia, and circulatory disorders. It appears to be very useful in older patients to increase blood flow in the brain. This supports the clinical use of GBE to treat cognitive impairment in the elderly. There are no reports on the transfer of GBE into breastmilk. So far, with exception of the seeds, GBE appears relatively harmless.

Relative infant dose:
Time to clear:
Lactation risk category: L3
Pregnancy risk category:
Adult dose:
Alternatives:

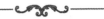

GINSENG

Trade names: Panax, Minomycin, Red Kooga

AAP recommendation: Not reviewed

Ginseng is perhaps the most popular and widely recognized herbal product. Early claims suggested that ginseng provided "strengthening" effects including increased mental capacity for work. A number of studies, mostly small and poorly controlled, have been reported. Many suggest helpful effects of ginseng with few side effects. Reported side effects include estrogen-like effects like nodules in the breast and vaginal bleeding, nervousness, excitation, morning diarrhea, and inability to focus. There are no reports on the transfer of ginseng into breastmilk, and we do not know if it is safe to use routinely in breastfeeding women.

Relative infant dose:
Time to clear:
Lactation risk category: L3
Pregnancy risk category:
Adult dose:
Alternatives:

GLATIRAMER

Trade names: Copaxone
AAP recommendation: Not reviewed

Glatiramer is used to treat multiple sclerosis. There are no reports on its transfer into breastmilk, but it is very unlikely due to its chemical structure. It is not likely to be harmful even if taken by mouth.

Relative infant dose:
Time to clear:
Lactation risk category: L3
Pregnancy risk category: B
Adult dose: 20 milligrams injected under the skin once daily
Alternatives:

GLIMEPIRIDE

Trade names: Amaryl
AAP recommendation: Not reviewed

Glimepiride is used to treat non-insulin dependent diabetes mellitis. There are no reports on the transfer of glimepiride into breastmilk. Caution is urged if used in breastfeeding women. Observe infant for low blood glucose levels.

Relative infant dose:
Time to clear: Between 24 and 45 hours
Lactation risk category: L4
Pregnancy risk category: B

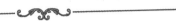

Adult dose: 1-4 milligrams daily
Alternatives:

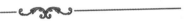

GLIPIZIDE

Trade names: Glucotrol XL, Glucotrol, Melizide, Minidiab,
Glibenese, Minodiab

AAP recommendation: Not reviewed

Glipizide is only used for the treatment of non-insulin-dependent (Type II) diabetes mellitus. No reports on the transfer into breastmilk were found. Other drugs in the same class as glipizide (tolbutamide, chlorpropamide) are known to pass into breastmilk in low amounts. Although low blood sugar in infants is a potential problem, no reports of this have been published. The new product, Metaglip, contains glipizide and metformin.

Relative infant dose:
Time to clear: Between 4.5 and 18.5 hours
Lactation risk category: L3
Pregnancy risk category: C
Adult dose: 15-40 milligrams daily
Alternatives:

GLUCOSAMINE

Trade names:

AAP recommendation: Not reviewed

Glucosamine is used to treat a form of arthritis. There are no reports on its transfer into breastmilk. However, it is very unlikely that glucosamine would enter breastmilk as the blood levels of glucosamine in the mother are extremely low. Further, its oral absorption is very low. It is, therefore, unlikely that an infant would receive harmful amounts of glucosamine.

Relative infant dose:
Time to clear: Between 1 and 1.5 hours
Lactation risk category: L3
Pregnancy risk category:
Adult dose:
Alternatives:

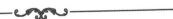

GLYBURIDE

Trade names: Micronase, Diabeta, Glynase, Glucovance, Euglucon, Gen-Glybe, Diaformin, Daonil

AAP recommendation: Not reviewed

Glyburide is used to treat non insulin-dependent (Type II) diabetes. Glyburide belongs to the sulfonylurea family (tolbutamide, glipizide) of drugs that lower blood glucose levels. Glyburide is one of the most potent in this family. Although there are no reports on the transfer of glyburide into breastmilk, others in this family are transferred into breastmilk in low levels. It appears that Glyburide does not even cross the placenta. Although we do not have reports of breastmilk levels, the levels are likely to be very low. The product, Glucovance, contains metformin and glyburide.

Relative infant dose:
Time to clear: Between 16 hours and 3 days
Lactation risk category: L3
Pregnancy risk category: B
Adult dose: 1.25-20 milligrams daily
Alternatives:

GLYCOPYRROLATE

Trade names: Robinul

AAP recommendation: Not reviewed

Glycopyrrolate is used before surgery as a drying agent. There are no reports on its transfer into breastmilk, but it is very unlikely that harmful amounts would transfer. Further, because glycopyrrolate is poorly absorbed after taken orally, it is unlikely that glycopyrrolate would pose a risk to a breastfeeding infant.

Relative infant dose:
Time to clear: Between 7 and 8.5 hours
Lactation risk category: L3
Pregnancy risk category: B
Adult dose: 1-2 milligrams three times daily
Alternatives:

GOSERELIN ACETATE IMPLANT

Trade names: Zoladex

AAP recommendation: Not reviewed

Goserelin is used to treat prostate cancer, endometriosis, and advanced breast cancer in premenopausal and perimenopausal women, among other uses. There are no reports on its transfer into breastmilk, but it is unlikely to enter breastmilk or to be absorbed orally by the breastfeeding infant.

Relative infant dose:
Time to clear: Between 9 and 11.5 hours
Lactation risk category: L3
Pregnancy risk category: X
Adult dose: 3.6 milligrams under the skin every 28 days.
Alternatives:

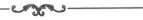

GRANISETRON

Trade names: Kytril

AAP recommendation: Not reviewed

Granisetron is a drug that prevents nausea and vomiting. It is commonly used with cancer chemotherapy. There are no reports on its transfer into breastmilk, but levels are likely to be low. Further, this family of drugs (see ondansetron) is not highly toxic and commonly used in children (2 years +) and pregnant women. It is unlikely that this product will be harmful to a breastfed infant. However, when used with chemotherapy drugs, the mother should not breastfeed until the chemotherapy drugs have cleared her system.

Relative infant dose:
Time to clear: Between 12 hours and 3 days
Lactation risk category: L3
Pregnancy risk category: B
Adult dose: 2 milligrams by mouth
Alternatives: Ondansetron

GREPAFLOXACIN

Trade names: Raxar

AAP recommendation: Not reviewed

Grepafloxacin is an antibiotic similar to ciprofloxacin. The manufacturer suggests that grepafloxacin was detectable in breastmilk after a 400 milligrams dose, but exact levels were not provided. Use grepafloxacin with caution, if at all, in breastfeeding women. See ciprofloxacin or ofloxacin as alternatives.

Relative infant dose:
Time to clear: Between 2.5 and 3.5 days
Lactation risk category: L4
Pregnancy risk category: C
Adult dose: 400-600 milligrams daily
Alternatives: Norfloxacin, Ofloxacin, Levofloxacin, Ciprofloxacin

GUAIFENESIN

Trade names: GG, Robitussin, Resyl, Benylin-E, Orthoxicol, Respenyl

AAP recommendation: Not reviewed

Guaifenesin is an expectorant used to loosen respiratory tract secretions. It does not suppress coughing and should not be used in persistent cough, such as smokers cough. There are no reports on its transfer into breastmilk. The poor usefulness of expectorants, in general, would suggest that breastfeeding mothers should not use them. However, no harmful effects have been reported in breastfeeding infants. Thus this product is probably quite safe for breastfeeding mothers, although it works poorly.

Relative infant dose:
Time to clear: Between 28 and 35 hours
Lactation risk category: L2
Pregnancy risk category: C
Adult dose: 200-400 milligrams every 4 hours
Alternatives:

GUANFACINE

Trade names: Tenex
AAP recommendation: Not reviewed

Guanfacine is used to treat high blood pressure and is similar to clonidine. There are no reports on the transfer of guafacine into breastmilk. Due to the potency of this product, caution is recommended in breastfeeding mothers.

Relative infant dose:
Time to clear: Between 3 and 3.5 days
Lactation risk category: L3
Pregnancy risk category: B
Adult dose: 1 milligram daily
Alternatives:

HALAZEPAM

Trade names: Paxipam
AAP recommendation: Not reviewed

Halazepam is used to treat anxiety disorders and is part of the valium family of drugs. Although no information is available on halazepam levels in breastmilk, its milk levels should be similar to that of diazepam. See diazepam.

Relative infant dose:
Time to clear: Between 2.5 and 3 days
Lactation risk category: L3
Pregnancy risk category: D
Adult dose: 20-40 milligrams three to four times daily
Alternatives: Alprazolam, Lorazepam

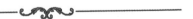

HALOPERIDOL

Trade names: Haldol, Novo-Peridol, Peridol, Serenace
AAP recommendation: Drug whose effect on nursing infants is unknown but may be of concern

Haloperidol is a potent antipsychotic agent. In one study of a woman receiving

5 milligrams twice daily, the amount of haloperidol in her breastmilk was very low. After 4 weeks of therapy, the infant showed no symptoms of sedation and was feeding well. Long-term exposure at higher levels might be slightly harmful in younger infants, but this is theoretical.

Relative infant dose: 2.5%
Time to clear: Between 2 and 8 days
Lactation risk category: L2
Pregnancy risk category: C
Adult dose: 0.5-5 milligrams two to three times daily
Alternatives:

HEPARIN

Trade names: Heparin, Canusal, Heplok, Pularin

AAP recommendation: Not reviewed

Heparin is used as an anticoagulant by injection because it is not orally absorbed. Heparin is very large in size and is very unlikely to transfer into breastmilk. Even if it were transferred to milk, it would rapidly be destroyed by the gastric content of the infant and would not be absorbed.

Relative infant dose:
Time to clear: Between 4 and 10 hours
Lactation risk category: L1
Pregnancy risk category: C
Adult dose: 4,000-5,000 units every 4 hours
Alternatives:

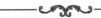

HEPATITIS A INFECTION

Trade names:

AAP recommendation: Maternal condition usually compatible with breastfeeding

Hepatitis A is an acute viral infection with symptoms of jaundice, fever, anorexia, and malaise (physical discomfort). In infants, the syndrome either has no symptoms or causes only mild, nonspecific symptoms. An injection of gamma globulin is the current therapy recommended following exposure to Hepatitis A. Nearly all adults are immune to Hepatitis A due to prior exposure.

Sudden and severe hepatitis A infection is rare in children and a carrier state is unknown. It is spread through fecal-oral contact and can be easily spread in day care centers. Viral shedding continues from onset up to 3 weeks. Unless the mother is acutely ill, breastfeeding can continue if the infant has had a gamma globulin injection. Proper hygiene should be stressed.

Relative infant dose:
Time to clear:
Lactation risk category:
Pregnancy risk category:
Adult dose:
Alternatives:

HEPATITIS B IMMUNE GLOBULIN

Trade names: H-BIG, Hep-B-Gammagee, Hyperhep

AAP recommendation:

Hepatitis B immune globulin (H-BIG) is a sterile solution of antibodies (10-18% protein) containing the antibody to the hepatitis B virus. It is most commonly used to treat infants born to hepatitis B positive mothers who wish to breastfeed. The infant should also be given the Hepatitis B vaccine (0.5 milliliters injected into the muscle) within 12 hours of birth, and again at 1 and 6 months.

Relative infant dose:
Time to clear:
Lactation risk category: L2
Pregnancy risk category: C
Adult dose: 0.06 milliliters per kilogram post-exposure X 3 over 6 weeks
Alternatives:

HEPATITIS B INFECTION

Trade names:

AAP recommendation: Not reviewed

Hepatitis B virus (HBV) causes a wide range of infections, ranging from no symptoms to sudden and severe fatal hepatitis. Chronic infections occur in 90% of infants who become infected during the birth process. Chronically infected individuals are at increased risk for chronic liver diseases and liver cancer in later life. HBV is transmitted through blood or body fluids. Hepatitis B proteins have been detected in breastmilk.

Infants of mothers who are HBV positive (HBsAg) should be given the

Hepatitis immune globulin (HBIG) within 1 hour of birth and a Hepatitis B vaccination at birth. This is believed to effectively reduce the risk of after birth transmission particularly by breastmilk. Several older studies have shown that breastfeeding poses no additional risk of transmission. So far, no cases of transmission of Hepatitis B by breastmilk have been reported following immunization of the infant.

Relative infant dose:
Time to clear:
Lactation risk category:
Pregnancy risk category:
Adult dose:
Alternatives:

HEPATITIS C INFECTION

Trade names:

AAP recommendation: Not reviewed

Hepatitis C (HCV) presents as a mild or no symptom infection with jaundice and malaise (physical discomfort). On average, 50% of the patients develop chronic liver disease, including cirrhosis of the liver and liver cancer in later life. HCV infection can be spread by blood to blood transmission; although most are transmitted by other unknown methods. Although transmission can occur during birth, this seldom happens.

Mothers infected with HCV could potentially transfer HCV by breastfeeding, but this has not been documented in a single case. The Center for Disease Control (CDC) does not consider chronic hepatitis C infection in the mother a reason not to breastfeed. The decision to breastfeed should be based largely on an informed discussion between the mother and her health care provider. Thus far, no confirmed case of HCV transmission has occurred from mother to child by breastfeeding.

Relative infant dose:
Time to clear:
Lactation risk category: L2
Pregnancy risk category:
Adult dose:
Alternatives:

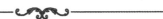

HERBAL TEAS

Trade names:

AAP recommendation: Not reviewed

Herbal teas should be used with great caution, if at all. A number of reports show harmful effects in pregnant women from some herbal teas which contain pyrrolizidine alkaloids (PA). Such alkaloids have been linked with destroying the fetus, birth defects, and liver toxicity. Other reports of severe liver toxicity requiring a liver transplant have occurred with an herbal antioxidant called "Chaparral".

A Chinese herbal product called "Jin Bu Huan" has been linked with hepatitis. Other remedies that are toxic to the liver include germander, comfrey, mistletoe, skullcap, margosa oil, mate tea, Gordolobo yerba tea, and pennyroyal (squawmint) oil. A recent report of seven poisonings following ingestion of "Paraguay Tea" suggests the tea contained other substances. A recent report on Blue Cohosh suggests it may cause heart problems when used late in pregnancy (see blue cohosh).

Because exact ingredients are seldom listed on many teas, this author strongly suggests that pregnant and breastfeeding mothers limit exposure to these substances as much as possible. Never consume herbal remedies if you don't know which herbs are in the tea. Remember, breastfeeding infants are much more susceptible to such toxins than adults.

Relative infant dose:
Time to clear:
Lactation risk category:
Pregnancy risk category:
Adult dose:
Alternatives:

HEROIN

Trade names:

AAP recommendation: Contraindicated by the American Academy of Pediatrics in breastfeeding mothers

Heroin, also known as diacetyl-morphine (diamorphine), is broken down to morphine. As a pain killer, morphine is generally considered an ideal choice for breastfeeding mothers when used postoperatively or for other forms of pain "in normal dosage ranges". Unfortunately, addicts and recreational users may use extraordinarily large doses of heroin. Heroin (morphine) is known to transfer into breastmilk. Large doses are likely to be very dangerous for a breastfed infant. Heavy users should probably not breastfeed and switch their infants to formula.

While it could be argued that recreational users could continue to breastfeed if they avoid doing so while under the influence of the heroin or prior to its use, this still may not be wise as it requires some understanding of the kinetics of morphine and its elimination. See morphine for more on its use.

Relative infant dose:
Time to clear: Between 6 and 10 hours
Lactation risk category: L5
Pregnancy risk category: B
Adult dose:
Alternatives:

HERPES SIMPLEX INFECTIONS

Trade names:

AAP recommendation: Breastfeeding is acceptable if no lesions are on the breast or are adequately covered

Herpes Simplex 1 and Herpes Simplex 2 have been isolated from breastmilk. Transmission after birth can occur and herpetic infections during the newborn period are often severe and fatal. Exposure to the virus from skin lesions of caregivers, including lesions on the breast, have been described. It is more likely for an infant to become infected during delivery than from breastmilk. Breastmilk does not appear to be a common mode of transmission. But, women with active lesions around the breast and nipple should not breastfeed from that breast unless the lesions are completely covered with bandages.

If the lesion is on the nipple or areola, pump and discard the milk from that breast until the lesion has healed. A number of cases of herpes simplex transmission via breastmilk have been reported. Women with active lesions should wash their hands carefully and often, to prevent spread of the disease from active lesions.

Relative infant dose:
Time to clear:
Lactation risk category:
Pregnancy risk category:
Adult dose:
Alternatives:

HEXACHLOROPHENE

Trade names: Septisol, Phisohex, Septi-soft, Sapoderm, Dermalex

AAP recommendation: Not reviewed

Hexachlorophene is an antibacterial agent. It is generally used topically as a surgical scrub and sometimes vaginally in mothers. Hexachlorophene is well absorbed through intact and denuded skin producing significant levels in the blood, brain, fat and other tissues in both adults and infants. It has been linked with causing brain lesions, blindness and respiratory failure in both animals and humans. Although there are no studies reporting amounts of this drug in breastmilk, it is probably transferred to some degree. This product should not be used on an infant's skin because it is highly absorbed and very harmful. Breastfeedng mothers should not use this product.

Relative infant dose:
Time to clear:
Lactation risk category: L4
Pregnancy risk category: C
Adult dose:
Alternatives:

HIV INFECTION

Common names: AIDS

AAP recommendation: Advise not to breastfeed

The AIDS (HIV) virus has been found in breastmilk. Recent reports from throughout the world have documented the transmission of HIV through breastmilk. At least 9 or more cases in the literature currently suggest that HIV-1 is secreted and can be transmitted to the infant via breastmilk. Although these studies show an obvious risk, currently no studies clearly show the exact risk associated with breastfeeding in HIV infected women. Women who develop a primary HIV infection while breastfeeding may shed very high levels of HIV virus and pose a high risk of transmission to their infants. HIV-infected mothers in the USA and others countries with safe alternative sources of feeding should be advised not to breastfeed their infants. Mothers at-risk for HIV should discuss this with their doctor prior to breastfeeding.

Relative infant dose:
Time to clear:
Lactation risk category: L5 in developed countries
Pregnancy risk category:
Adult dose:
Alternatives:

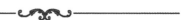

HYDRALAZINE

Trade names: Apresoline, Novo-Hylazin, Apo-Hydralazine, Alphapress

AAP recommendation: Maternal medication usually compatible with breastfeeding

Hydralazine is a popular antihypertensive used for severe high blood pressure during pregnancy and postpartum high blood pressure. It is transferred into breastmilk; although, the amount transferred to the infant would be too low to be harmful.

Relative infant dose: 1.2%
Time to clear: Between 6 hours and 1.5 days
Lactation risk category: L2
Pregnancy risk category: C
Adult dose: 10-25 milligrams four times daily
Alternatives:

HYDROCHLOROTHIAZIDE

Trade names: Hydrodiuril, Esidrix, Oretic, Diuchlor H, Novo-Hydrazide, Amizide, Dyazide, Modizide, Direma, Esidrex

AAP recommendation: Maternal medication usually compatible with breastfeeding

Hydrochlorothiazide (HCTZ) is a diuretic which acts by increasing the flow of urine. HCTZ is transferred into breastmilk in very small amounts. No HCTZ could be detected in the blood of a breastfeeding infant in one study. Although rare, it is thought that diuretics, in general, may decrease the volume of breastmilk. Some authors suggest that HCTZ can produce a reduction of blood platelets (thrombocytopenia) in the breastfeeding infant; although, this has not been proven. Most thiazide diuretics may be used when breastfeeding if doses are kept low.

Relative infant dose:
Time to clear: Between 22.5 hours and 3 days
Lactation risk category: L2
Pregnancy risk category: D
Adult dose: 25-100 milligrams daily
Alternatives:

HYDROCHLOROTHIAZIDE PLUS TRIAMTERENE

Trade names: Dyrenium, Maxzide, Novo-Triamzide, Dyazide, Hydrene

AAP recommendation: Not reviewed

Hydrochlorothiazide and triamterene are diuretics that increase urine production in humans. See the individual drugs.

Relative infant dose: 0.2%
Time to clear: Between 6 and 12.5 hours
Lactation risk category: L3
Pregnancy risk category: B
Adult dose: 25-50 milligrams hydrochlorothiazide (37.5-75 milligrams triamterene) daily.

Alternatives:

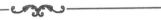

HYDROCODONE

Trade names: Lortab, Vicodin, Robidone, Hycomine, Actron

AAP recommendation: Not reviewed

Hydrocodone is a pain killer and relieves or suppresses coughs. It is structurally related to codeine; although, more potent. It is commonly used in breastfeeding mothers throughout the world. There are no reports on hydrocodone levels in breastmilk. To reduce exposure of the infant, feed the infant prior to taking the drug. Newborns may be more sensitive to this product so observe for sedation or constipation.

Most authors suggest that doses of 5 milligrams every 4 hours or more has a minimal effect on nursing infants, particularly in full term or older infants. However, prolonged use of higher doses could lead to sedation in the breastfed infant. Use sparingly.

Relative infant dose:
Time to clear: Between 15 and 19 hours
Lactation risk category: L3
Pregnancy risk category: B
Adult dose: 5-10 milligrams every 4-6 hours
Alternatives: Codeine

HYDROCORTISONE TOPICAL

Trade names: Westcort, Cortone, Emo-Cort, Aquacort,
Dermaid, Egocort, Hycor, Cortef, Dermacort

AAP recommendation: Not reviewed

Hydrocortisone is a steroid. When it is applied to the skin, it suppresses inflammation and enhances healing. The amount absorbed depends on the placement; 1% is absorbed from the forearm, 2% from the rectum, 4% from the scalp, 7% from the forehead, and 36% from the scrotal area. The amount transferred into breastmilk has not been reported, but as with most steroids, it is believed to be very small. Small amounts may be applied to the nipple for a few days only. Remove any unabsorbed or excessive ointment before breastfeeding. The 0.5% to 1% ointments are generally preferred to the creams. Use sparingly.

Relative infant dose:
Time to clear: Between 4 and 10 hours
Lactation risk category: L2
Pregnancy risk category: C
Adult dose: Apply topically four times daily
Alternatives:

HYDROQUINONE

Trade names: Esoterica, Eldoquin, Melpaque, Melanex,
Solaquin, Nuquin, Viquin

AAP recommendation: Not reviewed

Hydroquinone is used for depigmentation of the skin due to conditions such as freckles, melasma (discoloration of facial skin associated with pregnancy), senile lentigo (a brownish patch on the skin associated with old age and in people with sun-damaged skin), and inactive chloasma (tan discoloration of the skin associated with prenancy or the use of oral contraceptives). The amount absorbed by the skin is reported to be about 35%. This is high for topical preparations. Hydroquinone distributes rapidly and widely. There are no reports on the transfer of hydroquinone into breastmilk; although, some transfer is expected. While it does not seem to be very toxic, breastfeeding mothers should wait until after weaning to treat these skin conditions.

Relative infant dose:
Time to clear:
Lactation risk category: L3
Pregnancy risk category: C

Adult dose: Apply 2-4% solutions twice daily. Limit areas treated.
Alternatives:

HYDROXYCHLOROQUINE

Trade names: Plaquenil, Plaqueril

AAP recommendation: Maternal medication usually compatible with breastfeeding

Hydroxychloroquine (HCQ) is used to treat malaria and immune syndromes such as rheumatoid arthritis and Lupus erythematosus. HCQ is known to damage the retina (eye) if used for long periods, although this is rare. Patients on this product should probably see an eye doctor on a regular basis. HCQ is mostly broken down to form chloroquine. It has a very long half-life. See chloroquine. The pediatric dose for the prevention of malaria is 5 milligrams per kilogram per week which is far more than would be consumed via milk. Breastfeeding infants are unlikely to receive enough through breastmilk to cause eye problems.

Relative infant dose: 2.9%
Time to clear: Between 160 and 200 days
Lactation risk category: L2
Pregnancy risk category: C
Adult dose: 400 milligrams every week X 10 weeks
Alternatives:

HYDROXYZINE

Trade names: Atarax, Vistaril, Novo-Hydroxyzin

AAP recommendation: Not reviewed

Hydroxyzine is an antihistamine structurally similar to cyclizine and meclizine. It depresses the central nervous system (sedation), produces drying, and is used to treat nausea and vomiting. Hydroxyzine is largely broken down to form cetirizine (Zyrtec). There are no reports on the transfer of hydroxyzine into breastmilk. See cetirizine for a better alternative.

Relative infant dose:
Time to clear: Between 12 and 35 hours
Lactation risk category: L1
Pregnancy risk category: C
Adult dose: 50-100 milligrams four times daily

Alternatives: Cetirizine, Loratadine

HYOSCYAMINE

Trade names: Anaspaz, Levsin, NuLev, Buscopan,
                Hyoscine

AAP recommendation: Not reviewed

Hyoscyamine is a drug that dries secretions. Its side effects are constipation, dilated pupils, blurred vision, and urinary retention. Although exact amounts are not listed, hyoscyamine is known to transfer into breastmilk in trace amounts. So far, no harmful effects from breastfeeding while using hyoscyamine have been reported. In the past, Levsin (hyoscyamine) drops were used in infants for colic, but it is no longer recommended for this use.

As with atropine, infants and children are especially sensitive to this class of drugs (anticholinergics) and their use is sometimes discouraged. Although unreported, it is possible that this drug might impact milk supply, but this is remote. Use with caution.

Relative infant dose:
Time to clear: Between 14 and 17.5 hours
Lactation risk category: L3
Pregnancy risk category: C
Adult dose: 0.125-0.25 milligrams four times daily
Alternatives:

IBUPROFEN

Trade names: Advil, Nuprin, Motrin, Pediaprofen,
                Amersol, ACT-3, Brufen, Nurofen

AAP recommendation: Maternal medication usually compatible with
                breastfeeding

Ibuprofen is a nonsteroidal anti-inflammatory pain killer. It is often used for fever in infants. Ibuprofen enters milk in very low levels (less than 0.6% of maternal dose). Even large doses produce very small milk levels. Ibuprofen is an ideal pain killer for breastfeeding mothers.

Relative infant dose: 0.7%
Time to clear: Between 7 and 12.5 hours
Lactation risk category: L1

Pregnancy risk category: B in 1st and 2nd trimester
                              D in 3rd trimester
Adult dose: 400 milligrams every 4-6 hours
Alternatives: Acetaminophen

IMIPENEM-CILASTATIN

Trade names: Primaxin

AAP recommendation: Not reviewed

Imipenem is an antibiotic. Cilastatin is added to prevent imipenem from being broken down and inactivated. Both imipenem and cilastatin are poorly absorbed after taken by mouth and must be injected. There are no reports, but transfer into breastmilk is probably very low to nil. Changes in gastrointestinal flora could occur, but this is unlikely.

Relative infant dose:
Time to clear: Between 3.5 and 6.5 hours
Lactation risk category: L2
Pregnancy risk category: C
Adult dose: 500-750 milligrams twice daily
Alternatives:

IMIPRAMINE

Trade names: Tofranil, Janimine, Impril, Novo-Pramine,
                 Melipramine, Tofanil

AAP recommendation: Drug whose effect on nursing infants is
                        unknown but may be of concern

Imipramine is an antidepressant. It is transferred into breastmilk in small amounts. An infant would likely ingest about 0.2 milligrams per liter of milk. The long half-life of imipramine in infants could, under certain conditions, lead to high blood levels, but this has not been reported. Although no harmful effects have been reported, the infant should be monitored closely.

Relative infant dose: 0.2%
Time to clear: Between 1 and 3.5 days
Lactation risk category: L2
Pregnancy risk category: D
Adult dose: 75-100 milligrams daily

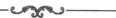

Alternatives: Amoxapine

INSULIN

Trade names: Humulin, Humalog, Iletin, Mixtard, Protaphane, Monotard

AAP recommendation: Not reviewed

Only small amounts of insulin are present in milk, probably by leakage from the mothers' blood supply. Even if it were present in significant amounts, it would be destroyed in the infant gut before being absorbed. The use of insulin by breastfeeding mothers is safe.

Relative infant dose:
Time to clear:
Lactation risk category: L1
Pregnancy risk category: B
Adult dose:
Alternatives:

IODINATED GLYCEROL

Trade names: Organidin, Iophen, R-GEN, Organidin

AAP recommendation: Not reviewed

Iodinated glycerol contains 50% organically bound iodine. High levels of iodine are known to be secreted in breastmilk and could suppress thyroid function in the infant. Normal iodine levels in breastmilk are already four times higher than the recommended dietary allowance (RDA) for infants. For some years, many iodine-containing cough products have been replaced with guaifenesin which is thought to be much safer. High levels of iodine-containing drugs, including this product, should not be used in breastfeeding mothers.

Relative infant dose:
Time to clear:
Lactation risk category: L4
Pregnancy risk category: X
Adult dose:
Alternatives:

IPRATROPIUM BROMIDE

Trade names: Atrovent, Apo-Ipravent

AAP recommendation: Not reviewed

Ipratropium is inhaled into the lungs to treat asthma. Although there are no reports, it probably transfers into breastmilk in extraordinarily low levels. It is unlikely that the infant would absorb any of this drug from breastfeeding due to the poor absorption of this family of drugs.

Relative infant dose:
Time to clear: Between 8 and 10 hours
Lactation risk category: L2
Pregnancy risk category: B
Adult dose: 36 micrograms four times daily
Alternatives:

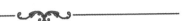

IRON

Trade names: Fer-In-Sol, Jectofer, Slow-Fe, Feospan

AAP recommendation: Not reviewed

The secretion of iron salts into breastmilk appears to be very low even following high maternal doses. However, while only small amounts of iron are transferred into milk, that present in human milk is highly absorbable by the infant. Premature infants are more likely to have iron deficiencies because their livers do not contain as high levels of iron as found in full term infants. Many pediatricians recommend iron supplementation, particularly in exclusively breastfed infants, beginning at 6 months of age; although, this is controversial. Supplementation in pre-term infants should probably be started earlier. Again, avoid very high doses.

Relative infant dose:
Time to clear:
Lactation risk category: L1
Pregnancy risk category:
Adult dose: 50-100 milligrams three times daily
Alternatives:

IRON DEXTRAN

Trade names: InFed

AAP recommendation: Not reviewed

Iron dextran is a solution of ferric hydroxide and dextran. It is available as an injection. It is used for severe iron deficiency anemia. While there are no reports on the transfer of iron dextran into breastmilk, it is very unlikely. It is well known that dietary supplements of iron do not significantly change the levels of iron in breastmilk. Pregnant moms please note: while the pregnancy risk category is only C, it has been shown to cause fetal deformaties in other species. Great care should be used in pregnant women.

Relative infant dose:
Time to clear:
Lactation risk category: L2
Pregnancy risk category: C
Adult dose:
Alternatives:

ISOMETHEPTENE MUCATE

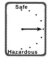

Trade names: Midrin

AAP recommendation: Not reviewed

Isometheptene is used in the management of tension and migraine headaches. The product "Midrin" also contains acetaminophen and a mild sedative, dichloralphenazone, of which little is known. No information is available on the transfer of isometheptene into breastmilk, but it is likely to attain low to moderate levels in breastmilk. Because better drugs exist for migraine therapy, this product is probably not a good choice for breastfeeding mothers. See sumatriptan, amitriptyline, or propranolol as alternatives.

Relative infant dose:
Time to clear:
Lactation risk category: L3
Pregnancy risk category:
Adult dose:
Alternatives: Sumatriptan, Amitriptyline, Propranolol

ISONIAZID

Trade names: INH, Laniazid, PMS Isoniazid, Pycazide,
                   Rimifon

AAP recommendation: Maternal medication usually compatible with
                          breastfeeding

Isoniazid (INH) is primarily used to treat tuberculosis. Although INH is transferred into breastmilk, it was not measurable in the infant's serum, but was detected in the urine of several infants. It is secreted into breastmilk in quantities ranging from 0.75 to 2.3% of the mothers dose. Caution and close monitoring of infants for liver toxicity and neuritis (nerve inflammation) are recommended.

Relative infant dose: 13.5%
Time to clear: Between 4.5 and 15.5 hours
Lactation risk category: L3
Pregnancy risk category: C
Adult dose: 5 milligrams per kilogram per day
Alternatives:

ISOTRETINOIN

Trade names: Accutane, Isotrex, Accure, Roaccutane

AAP recommendation: Not reviewed

Isotretinoin is a synthetic derivative of the Vitamin A family (retinoids). Isotretinoin is known to be incredibly teratogenic (can cause fetal deformaties) producing profound birth defects in exposed fetuses. It is primarily used for the treatment of acne. Transfer into breastmilk is unknown, but is likely as with other members of this family of drugs. Isotretinoin is extremely lipid soluble and concentrations in milk may be significant. The manufacturer strongly recommends that pregnant and breastfeeding mothers not use isotretinoin.

Relative infant dose:
Time to clear: Between 3.5 and 4 days
Lactation risk category: L5
Pregnancy risk category: X
Adult dose: 0.5-2 milligrams per kilogram per day
Alternatives:

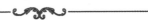

ITRACONAZOLE

Trade names: Sporanox

AAP recommendation: Not reviewed

Itraconazole is a drug used to treat fungal infections. Itraconazole is transferred into breastmilk at low levels. Its oral absorption by an infant is somewhat unlikely as it requires an acidic environment for absorption, unlikely in a diet high in milk. Itraconazole is not cleared for pediatric use. Until further studies are available, fluconazole is probably a preferred antifungal in breastfeeding mothers.

Relative infant dose: 0.2%
Time to clear: Between 10.5 and 13.5 days
Lactation risk category: L2
Pregnancy risk category: C
Adult dose: 200-400 milligrams daily
Alternatives: Fluconazole

KAOLIN - PECTIN

Trade names: Kaolin, Kaopectate, Kao-Con

AAP recommendation: Not reviewed

Kaolin and pectin (attapulgite) are used as antidiarrhea agents. Kaolin and pectin are not absorbed following oral use. Some preparations may contain opiate compounds and atropine-like substances, so check the bottle for other ingredients. Never use in children less than 3 years of age, but it is probably quite safe for breastfeeding mothers.

Relative infant dose:
Time to clear:
Lactation risk category: L1
Pregnancy risk category: C
Adult dose: 60-120 milliliters as needed
Alternatives:

KAVA-KAVA

Trade names: Awa, Kew, Tonga

AAP recommendation: Not reviewed

Kava-kava, also known as Kava, is the dried rhizome (plant stem) and roots of Piper methysticum. While more than 20 varieties are known, the black and white grades are most popular. Kava drink is prepared from the rhizome by steeping the pulverized root in hot water. It is then filtered and drunk. It is indigenous to the islands of the South Pacific where it is used like alcohol to induce relaxation. When chewed, kava induces a local anesthetic effect in the mouth. It is not known with certainty how these agents work, but they do induce sleep and reduce anxiety.

In humans, kava produces mild euphoria, happiness, and fluent, lively speech. High doses may lead to muscle weakness and vision and hearing changes. Heavy users are often underweight, have reduced plasma protein levels, facial edema, scaly rashes, elevated cholesterol, blood in the urine, elevated red blood cells, reduced platelets, and lymphocytes. Discolored, flaky skin and reddened eyes are common. Alcohol dramatically increases the toxicity of kava. Alcohol and Kava should not be used together. No information is available on the use of kava in pregnant or breastfeeding mothers, but it should be considered absolutely contraindicated. The German Commission E monographs state that it is contraindicated in pregnant and lactating women.

Relative infant dose:

Time to clear:

Lactation risk category: L5

Pregnancy risk category:

Adult dose:

Alternatives:

KETOCONAZOLE

Trade names: Nizoral Shampoo

AAP recommendation: Maternal medication usually compatible with breastfeeding

Ketoconazole is an antifungal agent that can be administered orally, topically and via shampoo. Ketoconazole is not detected in plasma after long-term use of the shampoo. Ketoconazole requires acidic conditions to be absorbed. Its absorption and distribution in children is not known. The oral absorption of ketoconazole varies and could be reduced in infants due to the alkaline condition induced by milk ingestion. Regardless, ketoconazole is probably safe in breastfeeding mothers with proper medical followup.

Relative infant dose: 0.4%
Time to clear: Between 8 and 40 hours
Lactation risk category: L2
Pregnancy risk category: C
Adult dose: 200-400 milligrams daily
Alternatives: Fluconazole

KETOPROFEN

Trade names: Orudis, Oruvail, Rhodis, Rhovail

AAP recommendation: Not reviewed

Ketoprofen is a typical nonsteroidal pain killer similar to ibuprofen. There is no information available on levels produced in breastmilk. See ibuprofen as alternative.

Relative infant dose:
Time to clear: Between 8 and 20 hours
Lactation risk category: L3
Pregnancy risk category: B
Adult dose: 50-75 milligrams three to four times daily
Alternatives: Ibuprofen

KETOROLAC

Trade names: Toradol, Acular

AAP recommendation: Maternal medication usually compatible with breastfeeding

Ketorolac is a popular, nonsteroidal pain killer used following surgery. Although previously used during delivery, it is used less frequently because it is believed to adversely affect fetal circulation and inhibit uterine contractions, increasing the risk of hemorrhage (bleeding). However, in one study of breastfeeding mothers, milk levels of ketorolac were not detectable in 4 of the subjects and was extremely low in the remaining milk samples. An infant would therefore receive less than 0.2% of the daily maternal dose. While it's use in postpartum mothers is controversial, it is minimally present in breastmilk and poses no risk to the breastfed infant.

Relative infant dose: < 0.2%

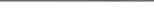

Time to clear: Between 9.5 hours and 2 days
Lactation risk category: L2
Pregnancy risk category: C in 1st and 2nd trimester
D in 3rd trimester
Adult dose: 30 milligrams every 6 hours
Alternatives: Ibuprofen

LABETALOL

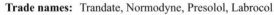

Trade names: Trandate, Normodyne, Presolol, Labrocol

AAP recommendation: Maternal medication usually compatible with breastfeeding

Labetalol is used in the treatment of hypertension (high blood pressure) and for treating angina pectoris (heart cramps). Only small amounts of labetolol are secreted into breastmilk. In one study of 3 breastfeeding women, milk levels were quite low. Measurable plasma levels were found in only one infant.

Relative infant dose: 0.6%
Time to clear: Between 1 and 1.5 days
Lactation risk category: L2
Pregnancy risk category: C
Adult dose: 200-400 milligrams twice daily
Alternatives: Propranolol, Metoprolol

LAMOTRIGINE

Trade names: Lamictal

AAP recommendation: Drug whose effect on nursing infants is unknown but may be of concern

Lamotrigine is a new anticonvulsant primarily indicated for treatment of seizures. Lamotrigine is transferred into breastmilk at moderate levels. In one study, the estimated daily dose to an infant would be 0.5 milligrams per kilogram per day and the plasma levels in infants were approximately 30% of the mothers plasma levels. Although the breastfeeding infant develops normally and no ill effects were noted, the blood levels of lamotrigine should probably be monitored periodically.

Relative infant dose: 22.8%
Time to clear: Between 5 and 6 days

Lactation risk category: L3
Pregnancy risk category: C
Adult dose: 150-250 milligrams twice daily
Alternatives:

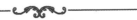

LANSOPRAZOLE

Trade names: Prevacid, PrevPac, Prevacid NapraPak,
Zoton

AAP recommendation: Not reviewed

Lansoprazole is used in the treatment of adult reflux and for the symptomatic relief of duodenal and gastric ulcers, among other uses. Lansoprazole is structurally similar to omeprazole. It is very unstable in stomach acid and largely denatured by the acidity of the infant's stomach. Although there are no studies of lansoprazole in breastfeeding mothers, its transfer to milk is likely low. Further, its oral absorption (via milk) is likely to be minimal in a breastfed infant as well. The only likely untoward effect would be reduced stomach acidity in the breastfeeding infant.

This product has no current pediatric indications; although, it is occasionally used in severe cases of erosive stomach inflammation. The product Prevpac contains Lansoprazole, Amoxicillin, and Clarithromycin.

Relative infant dose:
Time to clear: Between 6 and 7.5 hours
Lactation risk category: L3
Pregnancy risk category: B
Adult dose: 15-30 milligrams three times daily
Alternatives: Omeprazole, Famotidine

LEAD

Trade names:

AAP recommendation: Not reviewed

Lead is an environmental pollutant. It serves no useful purpose in the body and tends to accumulate in the body's bony structures. Due to the rapid development of the nervous system, children are particularly sensitive to elevated levels of lead. Lead apparently transfers into breastmilk at a rate proportional to maternal blood levels, but the absolute degree of transfer is controversial. Lead poisoning is known to significantly alter IQ and brain development, particularly in infants. Therefore, infants receiving breastmilk from mothers with high lead levels should be closely monitored.

Both mother and infant may require chelation therapy and the infant may need to be transferred to formula. Depending on the choice of chelator, mothers undergoing chelation therapy to remove lead may mobilize significant quantities of lead into their systems. They should not breastfeed during the treatment period unless the chelator is Succimer.

Relative infant dose:
Time to clear: Between 80 and 150 years
Lactation risk category: L5
Pregnancy risk category:
Adult dose:
Alternatives:

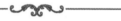

LEUPROLIDE ACETATE

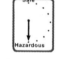

Trade names: Lupron, Viadur, Prostap
AAP recommendation: Not reviewed

Leuprolide is used in the management of endometriosis and as treatment of advanced prostate cancer, among other uses. Although leuprolide is contraindicated in pregnant women, no reported birth defects have been reported in humans. It is commonly used prior to fertilization, but should never be used during pregnancy. It is not known whether leuprolide transfers into breastmilk, but it is unlikely that its transfer would be extensive. Due to its extremely low oral bioavailability, it is unlikely that the breastfeeding infant would absorb much from breastmilk, even if it were present.

The effect of leuprolide on lactation is unknown, but it may suppress milk production particularly if taken during the early postpartum period. One study of a mother with high prolactin levels showed significant suppression of the milk hormone, prolactin, which is the reason for the L5 risk categorization. It is of no risk to the breastfed infant, only to milk production.

Relative infant dose:
Time to clear: Between 14.5 and 18 hours
Lactation risk category: L5
Pregnancy risk category: X
Adult dose: 3.75 milligrams every month
Alternatives:

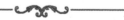

LEVALBUTEROL

Trade names: Xopenex

AAP recommendation: Not reviewed

Levalbuterol is the active form of albuterol. It is a popular bronchodilator used in asthmatics. No information is available on breastmilk levels. After inhalation, plasma levels are incredibly low. It is very unlikely that enough would enter breastmilk to produce clinical effects in an infant. This product is commonly used in infancy for asthma and other bronchoconstrictive illnesses.

Relative infant dose:
Time to clear: Between 13 and 16.5 hours
Lactation risk category: L2
Pregnancy risk category: C
Adult dose: 0.63 milligrams every 6-8 hours by nebulization
Alternatives:

LEVETIRACETAM

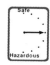

Trade names: Keppra

AAP recommendation: Not reviewed

Levetiracetam is an anticonvulsive agent. No data is available on the transfer of levetiracetam into breastmilk. Considering the chemical and physical properties of levetriacetam, breastmilk levels are probably moderate. Although this product is popular because of limited side effects, some caution is recommended until more information is available.

Relative infant dose:
Time to clear: Between 1 and 1.5 days
Lactation risk category: L3
Pregnancy risk category: C
Adult dose: 1000 - 3000 milligrams daily
Alternatives:

LEVOCABASTINE

Trade names: Livostin

AAP recommendation: Not reviewed

Levocabastine is an antihistamine primarily used in nasal sprays and eye drops. It is used for allergies affecting the eyes and nose. After application to the eye or nose, very low levels are absorbed and are too low to be clinically relevant in a breastfeeding mother or her infant.

Relative infant dose:
Time to clear: Between 5.5 and 8.5 days
Lactation risk category: L2
Pregnancy risk category: C
Adult dose: 1 drop four times daily
Alternatives:

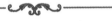

LEVOFLOXACIN

Trade names: Levaquin, Quixin

AAP recommendation: Not reviewed

Levofloxacin is the active ingredient in ofloxacin and its milk levels should be similar. See the report for ofloxacin for milk levels. The use of this family is increasing in pediatrics due to minimal toxicity.

Relative infant dose:
Time to clear: Between 1 and 1.5 days
Lactation risk category: L3
Pregnancy risk category: C
Adult dose: 500 milligrams daily
Alternatives: Norfloxacin, Ofloxacin

LEVONORGESTREL

Trade names: Norplant, Seasonale, Mirena, Triquilar,
                Levelen, Microlut, Microval, Norgeston

AAP recommendation: Maternal medication usually compatible with
                            breastfeeding

Levonorgestrel (LNG) is the active progestin in Norplant, Seasonale, and Mirena. From several studies, levonorgestrel appears to produce limited, if any, effect on breastmilk volume or quality. The level of progestin in the infant is approximately 10% that of maternal circulation. The sexual development of children exposed via breastmilk to trace levels of LNG is normal. The plasma concentration of levonorgestrel produced by Mirena are even lower than those produced by LNG contraceptive implants and with oral contraceptives. Because Mirena produces even lower plasma levels of this progestin, it is probably less likely to affect milk production than oral or implantable forms of progestins.

The new oral contraceptive Seasonale is an oral contraceptive that contains both levonorgestrel and the estrogen, ethinyl estradiol. It is used continuously for a three month period followed by withdrawal and menstruation. Due to its estrogen content, caution is recommended in breastfeeding mothers due to potential reduced breastmilk supply.

Relative infant dose:
Time to clear: Between 2 and 9.5 days
Lactation risk category: L2
                                L3 for Seasonale
Pregnancy risk category: X
Adult dose: Six 36 milligrams capsules under the skin
Alternatives:

LEVONORGESTREL (Plan B)

Trade names: Plan B
AAP recommendation: Not reviewed

Levonorgestrel is a progestin that can be used as an emergency contraceptive. It is believed to act by preventing ovulation or fertilization. Plan B is an emergency contraceptive that can be used to prevent pregnancy following unprotected intercourse or a known or suspected contraceptive failure. It is not effective if the woman is already pregnant or once the process of implantation has begun. To obtain maximal effectiveness, the first tablet should be taken as soon as possible and within 72 hours of intercourse.

The second tablet should be taken 12 hour later. Once lactation is established, it is unlikley that one dose of this medication will affect milk production or the infant.

Relative infant dose:
Time to clear: Between 2 and 9.5 days
Lactation risk category: L2
Pregnancy risk category:

Adult dose: 0.75 milligrams (one tablet) initially followed by a second tablet after 12 hours.

Alternatives:

LEVONORGESTREL AND ETHINYL ESTRADIOL (Preven)

Trade names: Preven

AAP recommendation: Not reviewed

Levonorgestrel and ethinyl estradiol (Preven) can be used as an emergency contraceptive to prevent pregnancy following unprotected intercourse or a known or suspected contraceptive failure. It is not effective if the women is already pregnant or once the process of implantation has begun. Each tablet contains a specific amount of levonorgestrel and ethinyl estradiol. They should not be used in known or suspected pregnant women or in patients with pulmonary edema, ischemic heart disease, deep vein thrombosis, etc. The initial treatment of 2 tablets should be administered as soon as possible, but within 72 hours of unprotected intercourse.

This is followed by the second dose of 2 tablets 12 hours later. It is not likely that one dose of this medication will affect milk production or harm the infant, but this is not known for sure.

Relative infant dose:
Time to clear:
Lactation risk category: L3
Pregnancy risk category:
Adult dose: 2 tablets followed by 2 additional tablets after 12 hours.
Alternatives: Plan B

LEVOTHYROXINE

Trade names: Synthroid, Levothroid, Unithyroid, Eltroxin, Levoxyl, Thyroid, Oroxine

AAP recommendation: Maternal medication usually compatible with breastfeeding

Levothyroxine is the active thyroid hormone thyroxine. Most studies indicate that minimal levels of maternal thyroid are transferred into breastmilk and that the amount transferred is extremely low and insufficient to alter the infant's thyroid function. The amount secreted after supplementing a breastfeeding mother is highly controversial and numerous reports conflict.

It is generally recognized that some thyroxine will transfer into breastmilk, but the amount will be extremely low. Remember that supplementation with levothyroxine is designed to bring the mother back to normal thyroid levels which is equivalent to the normal breastfeeding female. Hence, the risk of using thyroxine is no different than the thryoid levels found in a normal mother. Another form of thyroid, Liothyronine (T3), appears to transfer into breastmilk in higher concentrations than levothyroxine (T4), but liothyronine is seldom used in clinical medicine.

Relative infant dose:
Time to clear: Between 24 and 35 days
Lactation risk category: L1
Pregnancy risk category: A
Adult dose: 75-125 micrograms daily
Alternatives:

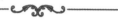

LIDOCAINE

Trade names: Xylocaine, Lignocaine, EMLA
AAP recommendation: Maternal medication usually compatible with breastfeeding

Lidocaine is a local anesthetic, sometimes used to treat heart arrhythmias. In at least 3 studies, the amount of lidocaine transferred into breastmilk was quite low. In addition, lidocaine is poorly absorbed when taken orally (by mouth) which will ensure low absorption in the breastfeeding infant. From studies performed, it is evident that a mother could continue to breastfeed while receiving local lidocaine injections or even lidocaine drips.

Relative infant dose: 2.9%
Time to clear: Between 7 and 9 hours
Lactation risk category: L2
Pregnancy risk category: C
Adult dose: 50-100 milligrams as needed
Alternatives:

LINDANE

Trade names: Kwell, G-well, Scabene, Kwellada, Quellada, PMS-Lindane, Desitan
AAP recommendation: Not reviewed

Lindane is an older pesticide also called gamma benzene hexachloride. It was formerly indicated for treatment of head lice and less so for scabies (crab lice). It is not recommended for use in neonates or young children at all. Lindane is transferred into breastmilk; although, the exact amounts have not been reported. The manufacturer estimates that the total amount of lindane an infant would receive from breastfeeding (30 micrograms per day) would probably be clinically insignificant. If used in children, lindane should not be left on the skin for more than 6 hours before being washed off.

Although there are reports of some resistance, head lice and scabies should generally be treated with permethrin products (NIX, Elimite) which are much safer in pediatric patients. See the monograph of permethrin.

Relative infant dose:
Time to clear: Between 3 and 4.5 days
Lactation risk category: L4
Pregnancy risk category: B
Adult dose: Topical
Alternatives:

LINEZOLID

Trade names: Zyvox
AAP recommendation: Not reviewed

Linezolid is an antibiotic. It is not known if linezolid is transferred into human milk, but levels will likely be quite low. Observe for changes in gut flora and diarrhea.

Relative infant dose:
Time to clear: Between 21 and 26 hours
Lactation risk category: L3
Pregnancy risk category: C
Adult dose: 400-600 milligrams every 12 hours
Alternatives:

LIOTHYRONINE

Trade names: Cytomel, Tertroxin
AAP recommendation: Not reviewed

Liothyronine is also called T3. It is infrequently used for thyroid replacement therapy. Although low levels of T3 are believed transported into milk, these levels are quite low. Mothers consuming liothyronine and thyroxine may breastfeed.

Relative infant dose:
Time to clear: Between 4 and 5 days
Lactation risk category: L2
Pregnancy risk category: A
Adult dose: 25-75 micrograms daily
Alternatives:

LISINOPRIL

Trade names: Prinivil, Zestril, Apo-Lisinopril, Carace

AAP recommendation: Not reviewed

Lisinopril is used in the management of hypertension. No breastfeeding data is available on lisinopril. See enalapril, benazepril, captopril as alternatives.

Relative infant dose:
Time to clear: Between 2 and 2.5 days
Lactation risk category: L3
Pregnancy risk category: D
Adult dose: 20-40 milligrams daily
Alternatives: Captopril, Enalapril

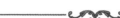

LITHIUM CARBONATE

Trade names: Lithobid, Eskalith, Duralith, Lithane,
                          Lithicarb, Camcolit, Liskonum, Phasal

AAP recommendation: Drug associated with significant side effects and
                          should be taken with caution

Lithium is a potent antimanic drug used in the management of bipolar disorders. Its use in the first trimester of pregnancy may be associated with a number of birth anomalies, particularly cardiovascular. Lithium is transferred into breastmilk at moderate to high levels and is absorbed by the breastfed infant. Some toxic effects have been reported. In one study, an infant exposed to lithium both during pregnancy and through breastfeeding was floppy, unresponsive and exhibited heart abnormalities which are indicative of lithium toxicity. Infants of breastfeeding mothers taking lithium should be closely monitored for blood lithium levels.

It takes at least 10 days for the infant's blood lithium levels to reach maximum concentration. Several studies of lithium use in breastfeeding mothers suggest that lithium administration is not an absolute contraindication to breastfeeding if the infant is monitored closely for elevated plasma lithium. Current studies, as well as unpublished experience, suggest that the infant's plasma levels rise to about 30-40% of the maternal level, most often without untoward effects in the infant.

However, numerous recent studies suggest that certain anticonvulsants such as valproic acid, lamotrigine, and others may be as effective as lithium in treating mania. These medications are probably safer to use in breastfeeding mothers.

Relative infant dose:
Time to clear: Between 3 and 5 days
Lactation risk category: L4
Pregnancy risk category: D
Adult dose: 600 milligrams three times daily
Alternatives: Valproic acid, Carbamazepine

LOPERAMIDE

Trade names: Imodium, Pepto diarrhea control,
                 Kaopectate II caplets, Maalox anti-diarrheal caplets,
                 Imodium Advanced, Novo-Loperamide, Gastro-Stop
AAP recommendation: Maternal medication usually compatible with
                         breastfeeding

Loperamide is an antidiarrheal drug. Because it is only minimally absorbed orally (0.3%), only small amounts are secreted into breastmilk. It is very unlikely that the reported levels of loperamide in breastmilk would ever produce clinical effects in a breastfed infant.

Relative infant dose: 0.03%
Time to clear: Between 43 and 54 hours
Lactation risk category: L2
Pregnancy risk category: B
Adult dose: 4 milligrams as needed
Alternatives:

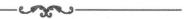

LORATADINE

Trade names: Claritin, Claratyne, Clarityn

AAP recommendation: Maternal medication usually compatible with breastfeeding

Loratadine is a long-acting antihistamine with minimal sedative properties. In one study, only 0.01% of the administered dose was transferred into breastmilk after 48 hours. It is very unlikely this dose would present a hazard to infants. In another study, the infant only received 0.46% of the loratadine dose received by the mother. It is very unlikely this dose would present a hazard to infants. Loratadine does not transfer into the brain of adults, so it is unlikely to induce sedation in infants. Pediatric formulations of loratadine are available.

Relative infant dose: 0.6%
Time to clear: Between 1.5 and 6 days
Lactation risk category: L1
Pregnancy risk category: B
Adult dose: 10 milligrams daily
Alternatives: Cetirizine

LORAZEPAM

Trade names: Ativan, Novo-Lorazepam, Almazine

AAP recommendation: Drug whose effect on nursing infants is unknown but may be of concern

Lorazepam is part of the Valium family and is frequently used prenatally and presurgically as a sedative agent (sleeping aid). In one prenatal study, it was found to produce a high rate of depressed respiration, hypothermia (low body temperature) and feeding problems in newborns. In all of the studies that evaluated the level of lorazepam in breastmilk, it appeared that the amount of lorazepam transferred into breastmilk would be clinically insignificant. Mothers with infants who breath poorly should not use this product.

Relative infant dose: 2.5%
Time to clear: Between 2 and 2.5 days
Lactation risk category: L3
Pregnancy risk category: D
Adult dose: 1-3 milligrams two to three times daily
Alternatives: Midazolam

LOSARTAN

Trade names: Cozaar, Hyzaar

AAP recommendation: Not reviewed

Losartan is used in the management of hypertension. No data are available on the transfer of losartan into breastmilk. Although it significantly penetrates the central nervous system, its ability to enter breastmilk is probably minimal. This product is only intended for those few individuals who cannot take angiotensin-converting enzyme (ACE) inhibitors. The trade name Hyzaar contains losartan plus hydrochlorothiazide (diuretic).

Relative infant dose:
Time to clear: Between 16 and 45 hours
Lactation risk category: L3
Pregnancy risk category: C in 1st trimester
                              D in 2nd and 3rd trimester
Adult dose: 25-50 milligrams once to twice daily
Alternatives: Captopril, Enalapril

LSD

Trade names:

AAP recommendation: Not reviewed

LSD is a powerful hallucinogenic drug. No data are available on the transfer of LSD into breastmilk. However, due to its extreme potency and its ability to enter the brain, LSD is likely to penetrate breastmilk and produce hallucinogenic effects in the infant. This drug is definitely CONTRAINDICATED in breastfeeding mothers. Mothers should refrain from breastfeeding for at least 24 hours after taking LSD. Milk should be pumped and discarded.

Relative infant dose:
Time to clear: Approximately 24 hours
Lactation risk category: L5
Pregnancy risk category:
Adult dose:
Alternatives:

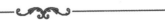

LYME DISEASE

Common names: Borrelia
AAP recommendation: Not reviewed

Lyme disease is caused by an infection with the bacterium, Borrelia Burgdorferi. This bacterium is transferred in-utero to the fetus and is secreted into breastmilk. It can cause infection in breastfed infants. If diagnosed postpartum or in a breastfeeding mother, the mother and infant should both be treated immediately. In breastfeeding patients, amoxicillin therapy is probably preferred. In the infant, amoxicillin with probenecid is preferred. Once treatment is initiated, mothers can resume breastfeeding.

Relative infant dose:
Time to clear:
Lactation risk category:
Pregnancy risk category:
Adult dose:
Alternatives:

LYSINE

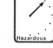

Common names: L-Lysine
AAP recommendation: Not reviewed

Lysine is a naturally occurring amino acid. The average American ingests from 6-10 grams daily in various foods. Aside from its use as a supplement in patients with poor nutrition, it is most often used for the treatment of recurrent herpes simplex infections. The risk of toxicity is considered quite low in both adults and infants. Rather high doses have been studied in infants as young as 4 months. Lysine is transferred into breastmilk; however, supplementation of breastfeeding mothers with L-lysine will probably not result in significantly elevated levels of free lysine in milk.

Only 0.54% of the administered dose of lysine was reported to be secreted into milk proteins. Further, the lysine present in milk was a protein, not free amino acids. Therefore, supplementation of breastfeeding mothers with L-lysine will probably not result in significantly elevated levels of free lysine in milk. More importantly, its usefulness is undocumented and probably limited, and it may not be worth the risk to the infant.

Relative infant dose:
Time to clear: Between 14.5 and 18.5 hours
Lactation risk category: L2
Pregnancy risk category:
Adult dose:

Alternatives:

MAGNESIUM HYDROXIDE

Trade names: Milk of Magnesia, Mylanta, Gastrobrom,
Phillip's Milk of Magnesia
AAP recommendation: Not reviewed

Magnesium hydroxide appears in laxative preparations and is poorly absorbed from maternal gastrointestinal tracts. Only about 15-30% of an orally ingested magnesium product is absorbed, the remaining stays in the gut and acts as a laxative. Magnesium rapidly deposits in bone (> 50%) and is significantly distributed to tissue sites. See the monograph of magnesium sulfate. It is unlikely to bother a breastfed infant.

Relative infant dose:
Time to clear:
Lactation risk category: L1
Pregnancy risk category: B
Adult dose: 5-30 milliliters as needed
Alternatives:

MAGNESIUM SULFATE

Trade names: Epsom salt, Magnoplasm, Salvital, Zinvit

AAP recommendation: Maternal medication usually compatible with breastfeeding

Magnesium is a normal blood electrolyte. It is used pre- and postnatally as an effective anticonvulsant in pre-eclamptic patients (a dangerous state of high blood pressure and fluid retention in pregnant women). One study indicated that magnesium is transferred into breastmilk, but only minimally above baseline levels. However, it is very unlikely that the amount of magnesium in breastmilk would be clinically relevant. In addition, the oral absorption of magnesium is very poor, averaging only 4-30%.

Relative infant dose: 0.2%
Time to clear: Between 12 and 15 hours
Lactation risk category: L1
Pregnancy risk category: B
Adult dose: 1-2 grams every 4-6 hours as needed

Alternatives:

MEBENDAZOLE

Trade names: Vermox, Sqworm
AAP recommendation: Not reviewed

Mebendazole is a medication used primarily for pin worms; although, it is active against round worms, hookworms and others. Mebendazole is poorly absorbed orally. Considering the poor oral absorption and high protein binding of mebendazole, it is unlikely that mebendazole would be transferred to the infant in clinically relevant concentrations. One case of reduced milk production has been reported in a mother who took 10 milligram twice daily for three days. Other studies did not report any change in milk production.

Relative infant dose:
Time to clear: Between 11 and 45 hours
Lactation risk category: L3
Pregnancy risk category: C
Adult dose: 100 milligrams twice daily
Alternatives: Pyrantel

MECLIZINE

Trade names: Antivert, Bonine, Ancolan, Sea-legs
AAP recommendation: Not reviewed

Meclizine is an antihistamine frequently used for nausea, vertigo and motion sickness; although, it is inferior to scopolamine. Meclizine was previously used for nausea and vomiting of pregnancy. No data are available on the transfer of meclizine into breastmilk. There are no pediatric indications for this product. This drug's usefulness is minimal and should probably not be used in breastfeeding mothers due to potential sedation in the infant.

Relative infant dose:
Time to clear: Between 24 and 30 hours
Lactation risk category: L3
Pregnancy risk category: B
Adult dose: 25-100 milligrams daily
Alternatives: Hydroxyzine, Cetirizine

MEDROXYPROGESTERONE

Trade names: Provera, Depo-Provera, Cycrin, Alti-MPA,
Gen-Medroxy, Farlutal, Provelle, Divina, Ralovera
AAP recommendation: Maternal medication usually compatible with
breastfeeding

Depo medroxyprogesterone (DMPA) is a synthetic progestin compound. It is commonly used for contraception when injected into the muscle. Due to its poor oral absorption, it is seldom taken orally. In a series of huge studies, the World Health Organization reviewed the developmental skills of children and their weight gain following exposure to progestin-only contraceptives during lactation. These studies documented that no adverse effects on overall development or rate of growth were notable. A number of other short and long-term studies available on development of children have found no differences with control groups.

Only small trace amounts of medroxyprogesterone (MPA) are transferred to breastfeeding infants and these amounts are not expected to have any influence on breastfeeding infants. It is well known that estrogens suppress milk production. With progestins such as this agent, it has been suggested that some women may experience a decline in milk production or poor early production following an injection of DMPA, particularly when the progestin is used early postpartum (12-48 hrs).

At present, there are no published data to support this nor is the relative incidence of this untoward effect known. Therefore, in some instances, it might be advisable to recommend treatment with oral progestin-only contraceptives first, so that postpartum women who experience reduced milk production could easily withdraw from the medication without significant loss of breast milk supply. Progestin contraceptives should not be used before at least 3 days postpartum and perhaps longer.

Relative infant dose:
Time to clear: Between 2.5 and 3 days
Lactation risk category: L1
                                              L4 if used first 3 days postpartum
Pregnancy risk category: D
Adult dose: 5-10 milligrams daily
Alternatives:

MEDROXYPROGESTERONE AND ESTRADIOL CYPIONATE

Trade names: Lunelle

AAP recommendation: Not reviewed

Lunelle is a new, once-a-month, injectable birth control product. It contains medroxyprogesterone acetate, which is the active ingredient in Depo-Provera and estradiol cypionate. The amount of medroxyprogesterone for this one month injection is 25 milligrams. The amount of Depo-Provera providing 3 months coverage is 150 milligrams. Because this injection contains estrogen, it may potentially reduce the production of milk and caution is recommended. Although small amounts of estrogens and progestins may pass into breastmilk, the effects of these hormones on an infant appear minimal.

Use of estrogen containing products, particularly during the early postpartum period, may dramatically reduce the volume of milk produced. Mothers should attempt to delay the use of these products for as long as possible postpartum (at least 6-8 weeks), if at all. Because of the estrogen content and the prolonged release formula, caution is recommended in breastfeeding mothers.

Relative infant dose:
Time to clear:
Lactation risk category: L3
Pregnancy risk category: X
Adult dose: 25 milligrams medroxyprogesterone, 5 milligrams estradiol cypionate monthly
Alternatives: Micronor, Ovrette

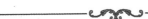

MELATONIN

Trade names:

AAP recommendation: Not reviewed

Melatonin (N-acetyl-5-methoxytryptamine) is a normal hormone secreted by a small gland in the human brain. Melatonin levels vary from night to day. It is believed that melatonin may induce a sleep-like pattern in humans, particularly at night. Some melatonin is known to pass into breastmilk and is believed to be responsible for training the newborn brain to shift its sleep-wake cycle to that of the mother. On average, the amount of melatonin in human milk is about 35% of the maternal plasma level, but can range as high as 80%.

After feeding breastmilk, melatonin levels appear to more closely reflect the maternal plasma level than prefeeding values, suggesting that melatonin may be transported into milk at night during the feeding rather than being stored in foremilk. In neonates, melatonin levels are low and progressively increase up to the age of 3 months. Night-time melatonin levels reach a maximum at the age of 1-3 years and then decline to adult values. The effect of orally administered melatonin on newborns is unknown, but melatonin has not been associated with significant harmful effects.

Relative infant dose:
Time to clear: Between 2 and 4 hours
Lactation risk category: L3
Pregnancy risk category:
Adult dose: 5 milligrams at bedtime
Alternatives:

MEPERIDINE

Trade names: Demerol, Pethidine

AAP recommendation: Maternal medication usually compatible with breastfeeding

Meperidine is a potent opiate pain killer. It is rapidly and completely broken down by the adult and neonatal liver to form normeperidine. Significant but small amounts of meperidine are transferred into breastmilk. Normeperidine has been detected in breastmilk up to 56 hours following a single dose of meperidine. One study clearly indicates that infants from mothers treated with meperidine (PCA post-cesarian) were neurobehaviorally depressed after three days. Infants from similar groups treated with morphine were not affected. Avoid meperidine while breastfeeding newborns.

Relative infant dose: 1.7%
Time to clear: Between 13 and 16 hours
Lactation risk category: L2
          L3 if used early postpartum
Pregnancy risk category: B
Adult dose: 50-100 milligrams every 3-4 hours as needed
Alternatives: Morphine, Fentanyl, Hydrocodone

MEPIVACAINE

Trade names: Carbocaine, Polocaine

AAP recommendation: Not reviewed

Mepivacaine is a long-acting local anesthetic similar to bupivacaine. Bupivacaine enters milk in exceedingly low levels. There are no reports on the transfer of mepivacaine into breastmilk; however, its structure is practically identical to bupivacaine so one would expect its entry into breastmilk to be low. Due to higher fetal levels and reported toxicities, mepivacaine is never used during delivery. Bupivacaine is preferred for use in breastfeeding women.

Relative infant dose:
Time to clear: Between 7.5 and 16 hours
Lactation risk category: L3
Pregnancy risk category: C
Adult dose: 50-300 milligrams once
Alternatives:

MERCURY

Trade names:

AAP recommendation: Not reviewed

Mercury is an environmental contaminant. Mercury poisoning produces brain damage, acute renal failure, severe gastrointestinal damage, and numerous other systemic toxicities. The amount of mercury that transfers into breastmilk depends on the form of mercury. The transfer of mercury into breastmilk is high at birth, then drops significantly at 2 months. Diet and mercury fillings are the most common sources of mercury. The amount of mercury in breastmilk is generally much higher in populations that eat large quantities of fish. Mercury from the diet is transferred into breastmilk at higher levels than mercury from older amalgam fillings.

The transfer of mercury from mercury fillings occurs mostly during pregnancy. The replacement of amalgam fillings should, if possible, be postponed until after pregnancy and breastfeeding. The removal of amalgam fillings while breastfeeding could potentially increase the release and transfer of mercury to the breastfed infant (this largely depends on the precautions taken by the dentist). Mothers known to have high levels of mercury should not breastfeed. Those with mercury-containing dental fillings should continue to breastfeed as the risk is minimal at this stage.

Relative infant dose:
Time to clear: Between 280 and 350 days
Lactation risk category: L5
Pregnancy risk category:
Adult dose:

Alternatives:

MESALAMINE

Trade names: Asacol, Pentasa, Rowasa, Canasa, Colazal,
Mesasal, Quintasa, Mesalazine
AAP recommendation: Should be given to nursing mothers with caution

Mesalamine is an anti-inflammatory agent used in ulcerative colitis. It contains 5-aminosalicylic acid, which is the active ingredient. 5-Aminosalicylic acid (5-ASA) can be converted into salicylic acid and absorbed, but the amount found in breastmilk is very small. The effect of mesalamine is primarily limited to the lining of the colon. Mesalamine is poorly absorbed from the gastrointestinal tract. Only 5-35% of a dose is absorbed. Oral tablets are enteric coated to ensure delayed absorption in the lower gut. The breastfeeding infant should be observed for diarrhea.

Relative infant dose: 8.8%
Time to clear: Between 20 and 50 hours
Lactation risk category: L3
Pregnancy risk category: B
Adult dose: 800 milligrams three times daily
Alternatives:

METAXALONE

Trade names: Skelaxin

AAP recommendation: Not reviewed

Metaxalone is a centrally-acting sedative used primarily as a muscle relaxant. Its ability to relax skeletal muscle is weak and is probably due to its sedative properties. Allergic reactions and liver toxicity have occurred in adults. There are no reports on the transfer of metaxalone into breastmilk.

Relative infant dose:
Time to clear: Between 8 and 15 hours
Lactation risk category: L3
Pregnancy risk category:
Adult dose: 800 milligrams three to four times daily
Alternatives:

METFORMIN

Trade names: Glucophage, Glucovance, Gen-Metformin, Glycon, Diaformin, Diabex, Diguanil, Glucphage

AAP recommendation: Not reviewed

Metformin belongs to the biguanide family. It is used to reduce glucose levels in non-insulin dependent diabetics (Type 2 diabetes mellitus). Metformin is transferred into breastmilk at very low levels. Plasma levels in infants were largely undetectable in several studies. No health problems were found in infants who were evaluated in one study. This product is now commonly used in pregnant patients and is probably safe for breastfeeding mothers and infants. The new product, Glucovance, contains metformin and glyburide. The new product, Metaglip, contains Glipizide and metformin.

Relative infant dose:	0.3%
Time to clear:	Between 25 and 31 hours
Lactation risk category:	L1
Pregnancy risk category:	B
Adult dose:	500 milligrams twice daily
Alternatives:	

METHADONE

Trade names: Dolophine, Physeptone, Biodone forte, Methex

AAP recommendation: Maternal medication usually compatible with breastfeeding

Methadone is a potent and very long-acting opiate pain killer. It is primarily used to prevent withdrawal in heroin addiction. Most studies show that only small amounts of methadone pass into breastmilk despite doses as high as 105 milligrams per day in the mother. About 2.8% of the maternal dose is believed to be transferred to the infant each day. Neonatal withdrawal syndromes are well known to occur in breastfeeding infants (exposed to methadone during pregnancy) following delivery. However, some methadone is transferred via milk and abrupt cessation of breastfeeding during high dose therapy has resulted in neonatal withdrawal in some infants. The Academy of Pediatrics recently placed methadone in the "approved" category for breastfeeding women.

Relative infant dose:	2.8%
Time to clear:	Between 2 and 11.5 days
Lactation risk category:	L3

Pregnancy risk category: B
Adult dose: 2.5-10 milligrams every 3-4 hours as needed
Alternatives:

METHICILLIN

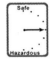

Trade names: Staphcillin, Celebenin, Metin, Celbenin

AAP recommendation: Not reviewed

Methicillin is a penicillin antibiotic. It is extremely unstable at acid pH (stomach), and it would therefore have limited oral absorption. There are no reports on the transfer of methicillin into breastmilk; although, it would appear to be similar to other penicillins. It is unlikely to be absorbed in a breastfeeding infant even if it penetrates the milk. Observe the infant for diarrhea.

Relative infant dose:
Time to clear: Between 4 and 10 hours
Lactation risk category: L3
Pregnancy risk category: B
Adult dose: 1 gram every 6 hours
Alternatives:

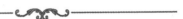

METHIMAZOLE

Trade names: Tapazole

AAP recommendation: Maternal medication usually compatible with
                        breastfeeding

Methimazole, carbimazole, and propylthiouracil are used to treat hyperthyroidism (over-active thyroid gland). Methimazole levels depend on the maternal dose, but appear too low to produce clinical effects in an infant. In two studies, no change was noted in the thyroid function of any infant, even when the maternal dose was high. Thus, using normal maternal doses, the authors suggest that methimazole should be considered safe for breastfeeding infants. However, during the first few months of therapy, the pediatrician should follow the infant closely for thyroid problems.

Relative infant dose: 1.5%
Time to clear: Between 1 and 3 days
Lactation risk category: L3
Pregnancy risk category: D

Adult dose: 5-30 milligrams daily
Alternatives: Propylthiouracil

METHOTREXATE

Trade names: Folex, Rhedumatrex, Ledertrexate,
                  Methoblastin, Arthitrex

AAP recommendation: Contraindicated by the American Academy of
                         Pediatrics in breastfeeding mothers

Methotrexate is a potent and potentially dangerous drug used in arthritic and other immunologic syndromes, among other uses. Methotrexate is secreted into breastmilk in small amounts. Authors from one study concluded that methotrexate therapy in breastfeeding mothers would not pose a problem for breastfeeding infants. However, methotrexate is believed to be retained in human tissue (particularly neonatal gastrointestinal cells and ovarian cells) for long periods (months).

One study has indicated a higher risk of fetal malformation in mothers who received methotrexate in the months prior to becoming pregnant. Therefore, pregnancy should be delayed for at least 3 months following therapy if either partner is receiving methotrexate. The concentration of methotrexate in breastmilk is minimal. However, due to the toxicity of this agent, it is probably wise to pump and discard the mother's milk (2-4 half-lives depending on the dose) after taking this product.

Relative infant dose: 0.1%
Time to clear: Between 1 and 1.5 days
Lactation risk category: L3 for acute use
                                L5 for chronic use
Pregnancy risk category: D
Adult dose: 10-30 milligrams
Alternatives:

METHYLDOPA

Trade names: Aldomet, Apo-Methyldopa, Dopamet,
                  Nova-Medopa, Aldopren, Hydopa, Nudopa

AAP recommendation: Maternal medication usually compatible with
                         breastfeeding

Alpha-methyldopa is a centrally-acting antihypertensive (an agent that reduces high blood pressure). It is frequently used to treat hypertension during pregnancy. Studies generally indicate that the levels of methyldopa transferred to a breastfeeding infant would be too low to be clinically relevant. However, gynecomastia (development of breasts) and galactorrhea (discharge of fluid from the nipple that looks like milk) has been reported in one full-term, two week old female neonate following seven days of maternal therapy with methyldopa, 250 milligrams three times daily.

In one study, the authors indicated that the maximum daily ingestion would be less than 855 micrograms or approximately 0.02 % of the maternal dose.

Relative infant dose: 0.1%
Time to clear: Between 7 and 9 hours
Lactation risk category: L2
Pregnancy risk category: C
Adult dose: 250-500 milligrams two to four times daily
Alternatives:

METHYLERGONOVINE

Trade names: Methergine, Ergometrine, Methylerometrine
AAP recommendation: Not reviewed

Methylergonovine is a drug used to control postpartum uterine bleeding. The ergots are powerful vasoconstrictors (an agent that causes the narrowing of blood vessels). Short-term (1 week), low-dose regimens of this drug does not seem to pose problems in nursing infants/mothers. In those situations requiring longer therapy, a risk/benefit assessment is required, but the drug is not likely to be overly hazardous to the infant. Methylergonovine is preferred over ergonovine because it does not inhibit lactation and levels in breastmilk are minimal.

Relative infant dose: 3.6%
Time to clear: Between 1.5 and 2.5 hours
Lactation risk category: L2
L4 for chronic use
Pregnancy risk category: C
Adult dose: 0.2-0.4 milligrams every 6-12 hours as needed
Alternatives:

METHYLPHENIDATE

Trade names: Ritalin, Concerta, Metadate CD, Methylin,
Metadate ER, Riphenidate, PMS-Methylphenidate

AAP recommendation: Not reviewed

The pharmacologic effects of methylphenidate are similar to those of amphetamines and include central nervous system stimulation. It is used for narcolepsy (recurring episodes of sleep during the day) and attention deficit hyperactivity disorder (ADHD). Methylphenidate is transferred into breastmilk, but the levels are quite low and no harmful effects have been reported in several breastfed infants. The risk of toxicity must be weighed against the need of mother and infant.

Relative infant dose: 1.9%
Time to clear: Between 4 and 15 hours
Lactation risk category: L3
Pregnancy risk category: C
Adult dose: 10 milligrams two to three times daily. Highly variable.
Alternatives:

METHYLPREDNISOLONE

Trade names: Solu-Medrol, Depo-Medrol, Medrol,
Advantan, Neo-Medrol

AAP recommendation: Maternal medication usually compatible with
breastfeeding

Methylprednisolone is a steroid. Used in normal doses, it would be very unlikely to affect a breastfed infant. But, the effect depends on dose and duration of exposure. For a complete description of steroid use in breastfeeding mothers see prednisone. In general, the amount of methylprednisolone and other steroids transferred into breastmilk is minimal as long as the dose does not exceed 80 milligrams per day. However, relating side effects of steroids received from breastmilk with the maternal dose is difficult. Each situation should be evaluated individually. Extended use of high doses could cause the infant to have steroid side effects including decreased linear growth rate (height). Low to moderate doses are believed to have minimal effects on breastfed infants. See prednisone.

Relative infant dose:
Time to clear: Between 11 and 14 hours
Lactation risk category: L2
Pregnancy risk category: C

Adult dose: 2-60 milligrams daily
Alternatives: Prednisone

METOCLOPRAMIDE

Trade names: Reglan, Emex, Maxeran, Maxolon, Pramin,
                   Gastromax, Paramid
AAP recommendation: Drug whose effect on nursing infants is
                          unknown but may be of concern

Metoclopramide has multiple functions, but is primarily used in GI reflux. Since 1981, a number of publications have documented major increases in breastmilk production following the use of metoclopramide, domperidone, or sulpiride. It is well recognized that metoclopramide increases a mother's milk supply in some cases, but it is exceedingly dose dependent and variable. Some mothers simply do not respond. Metoclopramide is commonly used (10 milligrams three times daily) to increase the milk supply by increasing the production of the milk hormone, prolactin. The transfer of metoclopramide into human milk is minimal, far less than the clinical doses used directly in infants. If this drug is used longer than 4 weeks, some mothers become depressed; although, some patients have used it successfully for months. If milk production is increased, the dose should be slowly decreased after it is well established. Do not abruptly stop this drug as your milk supply may suffer. Another dopamine antagonist, domperidone, is a preferred choice due to minimal side effects. Unfortunately, it is not available in the USA.

Relative infant dose: 4.4%
Time to clear: Between 20 and 30 hours
Lactation risk category: L2
Pregnancy risk category: B
Adult dose: 10-15 milligrams three times daily
Alternatives: Domperidone

METOPROLOL

Trade names: Toprol-XL, Lopressor, Betaloc,
                   Novo-Metoprol, Betaloc, Lopresor, Minax
AAP recommendation: Maternal medication usually compatible with
                          breastfeeding

Metoprolol is used to treat hypertension (high blood pressure), angina pectoris (heart cramps), and cardiac arrhythmias (disturbance of the heart rhythm). The absolute amount of metoprolol transferred to the infant is quite small. In a study of 9 women receiving 50-100 milligrams twice daily, the authors estimate the infant would receive 0.28 milligrams per day, an amount 20-40 times less than a typical clinical dose. Although these levels are too low to be clinically relevant, metoprolol should be used under close supervision.

Relative infant dose: 1.5%
Time to clear: Between 12 and 35 hours
Lactation risk category: L3
Pregnancy risk category: B
Adult dose: 100-450 milligrams daily
Alternatives: Propranolol

METRONIDAZOLE

Trade names: Flagyl, Metizol, Trikacide, Protostat, Noritate, NeoMetric, Novo-Nidazol, Metrozine, Rozex

AAP recommendation: Drug whose effect on nursing infants is unknown but may be of concern

Metronidazole is an antibiotic commonly used in infants and their mothers. While significant amounts are transferred into breastmilk, it is so safe that no harmful effects have been noted in any of the numerous infants studied. The authors estimated that the daily metronidazole dose received by the infant at 3.0 milligrams per kilogram with 500 milliliters milk intake per day, is well below the advocated 15-30 milligrams per kilogram recommended therapeutic dose for infants. The absorption of metronidazole from the vaginal gel, MetroGel, is minimal and would not likely enter milk in clinical ranges. When used in mothers at high doses (2 grams), breastmilk should be pumped and discarded for 12-24 hours.

Relative infant dose: 12.6%
Time to clear: Between 34 and 42.5 hours
Lactation risk category: L2
Pregnancy risk category: B
Adult dose: 250-500 milligrams twice daily
Alternatives:

METRONIDAZOLE TOPICAL GEL

Trade names: MetroGel Topical, Metrogyl, Metrogel

AAP recommendation: Not reviewed

Metronidazole topical gel is primarily indicated for acne and contains 0.75% metronidazole. See metronidazole. The topical application of metronidazole gel produces exceedingly low plasma levels in the mother and minimal to no levels in breastmilk.

Relative infant dose:
Time to clear: Between 34 and 42.5 hours
Lactation risk category: L3
Pregnancy risk category: B
Adult dose: Apply topically twice daily
Alternatives:

METRONIDAZOLE VAGINAL GEL

Trade names: Metrogel Vaginal, Metrogel

AAP recommendation: Drug whose effect on nursing infants is
                        unknown but may be of concern

Both topical and vaginal preparations of metronidazole contain only 0.75% metronidazole. Topical and intravaginal metronidazole gels are indicated for bacterial vaginosis. After using the drug, plasma levels are exceedingly low. Breastmilk levels following intravaginal use would probably be exceedingly low. The transfer of metronidazole into breastmilk may be lower for the gel than for vaginal preparations, primarily due to the low plasma levels attained with the gel.

Relative infant dose:
Time to clear: Between 34 and 42.5 hours
Lactation risk category: L2
Pregnancy risk category: B
Adult dose: 37.5 milligrams twice daily
Alternatives:

MICONAZOLE

Trade names: Monistat IV, Monistat 3, Monistat 7,
                Monistat, Daktarin, Daktozin, Fungo

AAP recommendation: Not reviewed

Miconazole is an effective antifungal that is commonly used intravenously, topically, and intravaginally. After topical application, there is little or no absorption (0.1%). Oral absorption of miconazole is poor, only 25-30%. After intravaginal application, approximately 1% of the dose is absorbed. It is unlikely that the limited absorption of miconazole from vaginal application would produce significant breastmilk levels. Breastmilk concentrations following oral and intravenous miconazole have not been reported. Miconazole is commonly used in pediatric patients less than 1 year of age.

Relative infant dose:
Time to clear: Between 1.5 and 5 days
Lactation risk category: L2
Pregnancy risk category: C
Adult dose: 200-1200 milligrams three times daily
Alternatives:

MIDAZOLAM

Trade names: Versed, Hypnovel

AAP recommendation: Effect on nursing infants unknown but may be of concern

Midazolam is a very short acting sedative that is used prior to surgery. The onset of action of midazolam is extremely rapid, its potency is greater than Valium (diazepam), and its elimination is very rapid. Midazolam was not found in milk 4 hours after the drug was taken. Therefore, the amount of midazolam transferred to an infant via early milk is minimal, particularly if the baby is breastfed more than 4 hours after the drug is taken.

Relative infant dose: 0.6%
Time to clear: Between 8 and 25 hours
Lactation risk category: L3
Pregnancy risk category: D
Adult dose: 1-2.5 milligrams once or twice
Alternatives: Lorazepam

MILK THISTLE

Common names: Holy Thistle, Lady Thistle, Silybum, Marian Thistle, Silymarin

AAP recommendation: Not reviewed

Milk Thistle is an herbal that has been used since 23 A.D. to protect the liver. Its main component, Silymarin, is believed to be a potent antioxidant and liver protective agent. Silymarin is poorly soluble in water so teas are ineffective. Only 23-47% is absorbed orally. Silymarin is believed to inhibit oxidative damage to cells and to stimulate the regenerative capacity of liver cells. While it has been advocated to increase milk supply, there is little evidence to show that it works.

There are no reports on the transfer of silymarin into breastmilk, but some probably transfers. However, the only reported side effects appear to be brief gastrointestinal intolerance and mild allergic reactions.

Relative infant dose:
Time to clear:
Lactation risk category: L3
Pregnancy risk category:
Adult dose: 200-400 milligrams daily via extracts
Alternatives:

MINOXIDIL

Trade names: Loniten, Minodyl, Rogaine, Apo-Gain,
                  Minox, Regaine

AAP recommendation: Maternal medication usually compatible with
                          breastfeeding

Minoxidil is a potent vasodilator (an agent that causes widening of blood vessels). It is used to treat hypertension, hair loss, and baldness. When applied topically to prevent hair loss, only 1.4% of the dose is absorbed. Long-term exposure of breastfeeding infants in women taking oral minoxidil may not be advisable. However, in those using topical minoxidil, the limited absorption by the skin would minimize blood levels and significantly reduce the risk of transfer to the infant via breastmilk. It is unlikely that the amount absorbed from topical application would produce clinically relevant amounts in breastmilk.

Relative infant dose: 7.7%
Time to clear: Between 14 and 21 hours
Lactation risk category: L2 topically
                               L3 orally
Pregnancy risk category: C
Adult dose: 10-40 milligrams daily
Alternatives:

MITOXANTRONE

Trade names: Novantrone, Onkotrone

AAP recommendation: Not reviewed

Mitoxantrone is an immune-suppressing agent used in the treatment of relapsing multiple sclerosis. Mitoxantrone is transferred into breastmilk. As this is a DNA-damaging agent that is distributed to many organs leading to prolonged plasma levels, it should not be used in breastfeeding mothers.

Relative infant dose:
Time to clear: Between 4 and 45 days
Lactation risk category: L5
Pregnancy risk category: D
Adult dose: 12 milligrams per meter squared
Alternatives:

MODAFINIL

Trade names: Provigil

AAP recommendation: Not reviewed

Modafinil is used in the treatment of narcolepsy (recurring episodes of sleep during the day) to help people stay awake. Although it is similar to amphetamines and methylphenidate (Ritalin), its method of action is unknown. There are no reports on its transfer into breastmilk. Some caution is recommended as its chemistry is ideal to enter breastmilk and may ultimately lead to higher milk levels.

Relative infant dose:
Time to clear: Between 2.5 and 3 days
Lactation risk category: L4
Pregnancy risk category: C
Adult dose: 200-400 milligrams up to twice daily
Alternatives:

MOMETASONE

Trade names: Elocon, Nasonex

AAP recommendation: Not reviewed

Mometasone is a steroid primarily intended for use in the nose and on the skin. It is considered a medium-potency steroid, similar to betamethasone and triamcinolone. Following topical application to the skin, less than 0.7% is absorbed over an 8 hour period. It is very unlikely that mometasone would be transferred into breastmilk in clinically relevant levels. Intranasal and topical applications are safe for breastfeeding mothers.

Relative infant dose:
Time to clear:
Lactation risk category: L3
Pregnancy risk category: C
Adult dose: Apply topically 2-3 times daily
Alternatives:

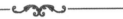

MONTELUKAST SODIUM

Trade names: Singulair

AAP recommendation: Not reveiwed

Montelukast is used in the treatment of asthma. There are no reports on the transfer of this drug into breastmilk. However, this product is cleared for use in children aged 6 and above, so it is not overly hazardous. Although milk levels in humans are unreported, they are probably quite low.

Relative infant dose:
Time to clear: Between 11 and 27.5 hours
Lactation risk category: L3
Pregnancy risk category: B
Adult dose: 10 milligrams daily
Alternatives: Zafirlukast

MORPHINE

Trade names: Duramorph, Infumorph, Morphitec, Statex,
M.O.S. MS Contin, Morphalgin, Ordine, Anamorph,
Kapanol, MS Contin, Oramorph, Sevredol

AAP recommendation: Maternal medication usually compatible with
breastfeeding

Morphine is a potent narcotic pain killer. Of the studies completed, most suggest the transfer of morphine into breastmilk is minimal at normal doses. One study performed in women who received morphine via patient-controlled analgesia (PCA) pumps for 12-48 hours postpartum, suggested that none of the infants were sedated at 3 days. When taken orally, morphine is poorly absorbed (26%) into the bloodstream. It is unlikely these levels would be clinically relevant in a stable breastfeeding infant. Infants under 1 month of age have decreased clearance of morphine compared to older infants. The clearance of morphine and its removal from the infant's system begins to approach adult values by 2 months of age.

Morphine is probably the preferred opiate in breastfeeding mothers. However, high doses over prolonged periods could lead to sedation and respiratory problems in newborn or premature infants.

Relative infant dose: 10.7%
Time to clear: Between 6 and 10 hours
Lactation risk category: L3
Pregnancy risk category: B
Adult dose: 10-30 milligrams every 4 hours as needed
Alternatives: Codeine

MOXIFLOXACIN

Trade names: Avelox, Vigamox
AAP recommendation: Not reviewed

Moxifloxacin is an antibiotic used orally, intravenously, and in the eye. There are no reports on its transfer into breastmilk. Ofloxacin or levofloxacin should be considered as alternatives until we have reports on this drug.

Relative infant dose:
Time to clear: Between 1.5 and 3.5 days
Lactation risk category: L2 ophthalmically
L3 orally, IV
Pregnancy risk category: C
Adult dose: Oral = 400 milligrams daily
Alternatives: Ofloxacin, Levofloxacin, Ciprofloxacin

MUPIROCIN OINTMENT

Trade names: Bactroban
AAP recommendation: Not reviewed

Mupirocin is a topical antibiotic used for impetigo (contagious skin infection), among other uses. Mupirocin is only minimally absorbed following topical application. The drug is absorbed orally, but it is so rapidly broken down that systemic levels are not sustained. It is quite safe for breastfeeding mothers, particularly on the infected nipple.

Relative infant dose:
Time to clear: Between 1 and 3 hours
Lactation risk category: L1
Pregnancy risk category: B
Adult dose: Apply sparingly
Alternatives:

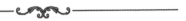

NABUMETONE

Trade names: Relafen, Relifex
AAP recommendation: Not reviewed

Nabumetone is a non-steroidal anti-inflammatory drug (NSAID) for arthritic pain. It is not known if the nabumetone metabolite (6MNA) is secreted into breastmilk. With the exception of ibuprofen and ketorolac, most NSAIDs are not generally recommended in breastfeeding mothers. See ibuprofen or celecoxib as an alternative.

Relative infant dose:
Time to clear: Between 3.5 and 6.5 days
Lactation risk category: L3
Pregnancy risk category: C
Adult dose: 500-1000 milligrams daily to twice daily
Alternatives: Ibuprofen

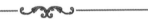

NADOLOL

Trade names: Corgard, Syn-Nadolol, Novo-Nadolol
AAP recommendation: Maternal medication usually compatible with
                         breastfeeding

Nadolol is used to treat high blood pressure. It is secreted into breastmilk in moderately high amounts. A 10 pound infant would receive from 2 to 7% of the maternal dose. The authors recommended caution with the use of this beta blocker in breastfeeding patients. Due to its long half-life and high milk/plasma ratio, this would not be a preferred beta blocker.

Relative infant dose: 4.7%

Time to clear: Between 3.5 and 5 days
Lactation risk category: L4
Pregnancy risk category: C
Adult dose: 40-80 milligrams daily
Alternatives: Propranolol, Metoprolol

NAFCILLIN

Trade names: Unipen, Nafcil
AAP recommendation: Not reviewed

Nafcillin is an intravenous antibiotic commonly used in infants. There are no reports on the levels of nafcillin in breastmilk, but it is likely to be small. Oral absorption in the infant would be minimal. Nafcillin is commonly used in infants to treat infections.

Relative infant dose:
Time to clear: Between 2 and 7.5 hours
Lactation risk category: L1
Pregnancy risk category: B
Adult dose: 250-1000 milligrams every 4-6 hours
Alternatives:

NALBUPHINE

Trade names: Nubain
AAP recommendation: Not reviewed

Nalbuphine is a potent narcotic pain killer similar in potency to morphine. According to the authors of one study, infants of mothers treated with 20 milligrams of nalbuphine did not show any measureable plasma concentrations.

Relative infant dose:
Time to clear: Between 20 and 25 hours
Lactation risk category: L2
Pregnancy risk category: B
Adult dose: 10-20 milligrams every 3-6 hours as needed
Alternatives:

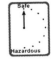

NALTREXONE

Trade names: ReVia, Nalorex

AAP recommendation: Not reviewed

Naltrexone is used in alcohol and heroin dependency. In a study of a patient receiving 50 milligrams per day, the infant achieved all expected milestones and showed no drug-related side effects. The infant only absorbed 0.86-1.06% of the mother's dose. Naltrexone was not found in the infants' plasma and levels of its break-down product were only marginally found.

Relative infant dose:	1.0%
Time to clear:	Between 16 hours and 3 days
Lactation risk category:	L1
Pregnancy risk category:	C
Adult dose:	50-150 milligrams daily
Alternatives:	

NAPROXEN

Trade names: Anaprox, Naprosyn, Aleve, Apo-Naproxen, Naxen, Inza, Proxen SR, Synflex

AAP recommendation: Maternal medication usually compatible with breastfeeding

Naproxen is a popular non-steroidal anti-inflammatory drug (NSAID) painkiller. Although the amount of naproxen transferred into the breastfeeding infant is minimal, it should be used with caution in nursing mothers because of its long half-life (time the active ingredient is in the body) and its effect on the infant's cardiovascular system, kidneys, and gastrointestinal tract. There is one reported case of prolonged bleeding and acute anemia in a seven-day-old infant. The relative infant dose was probably less than 3.3% of the mother's dose. Its short term use during the postpartum period or infrequent or occasional use later on would probably not affect the breastfeeding infant. Acetaminophen or Ibuprofen are preferred analgesics.

Relative infant dose:	3.3%
Time to clear:	Between 2 and 3 days
Lactation risk category:	L3
	L4 for chronic use
Pregnancy risk category:	B
Adult dose:	250-500 milligrams twice daily

Alternatives: Ibuprofen

NARATRIPTAN

Trade names: Amerge, Naramig
AAP recommendation: Not reviewed

Naratriptan is used to treat acute migraine headaches. There are no reports on the transfer of naratriptan into breastmilk. Naratriptan is a close relative of sumatriptan, only slightly better absorbed orally, and produces fewer side effects in sumatriptan-sensitive patients. Some studies suggest that sumatriptan is equal to if not more effective than naratriptan. Sumatriptan has been studied in breastfeeding mothers and produces minimal milk levels. See sumatriptan.

Relative infant dose:
Time to clear: Between 24 and 30 hours
Lactation risk category: L3
Pregnancy risk category: C
Adult dose: 1-2.5 milligrams every 4 hours X 2-3
Alternatives: Sumatriptan

NEFAZODONE HCL

Trade names: Serzone, Dutonin
AAP recommendation: Not reviewed

Nefazodone is an antidepressant similar to trazodone. In one study, a mother was taking 200 milligrams in the morning and 100 milligrams at night. Her 9 week old infant (5 lb) was admitted to the hospital with drowsiness, lethargy, failure to thrive, and poor temperature control. Since this infant was born premature at 27 weeks, these side effects may be due to immaturity. Nevertheless, this drug should probably not be used in breastfeeding mothers with young infants, premature infants, infants subject to apnea, or other weakened infants.

Relative infant dose: 1.3%
Time to clear: Between 4 and 20 hours
Lactation risk category: L4
Pregnancy risk category: C
Adult dose: 150-300 milligrams twice daily

Alternatives: Sertraline, Paroxetine, Trazodone

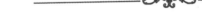

NICARDIPINE

Trade names: Cardene
AAP recommendation: Not reviewed

Nicardipine is structurally related to nifedipine. Animal studies indicate that it is secreted to some degree into breastmilk. There are no reports on breastmilk levels. See verapamil, nifedipine as better alternatives.

Relative infant dose:
Time to clear: Between 8 and 20 hours
Lactation risk category: L3
Pregnancy risk category: C
Adult dose: 5-15 milligrams every 1 hour as needed
Alternatives: Nifedipine, Nimodipine

NICOTINE PATCHES or GUM

Trade names: Habitrol, Nicoderm, Nicotrol, Prostep,
                Nicoderm, Nicorette, Nicotinell, Nicabate, Nicotinell TTS
AAP recommendation: Not reviewed

Nicotine and its break-down product, cotinine, are both present in breastmilk in significant concentrations. Earlier data suggested that cigarette smoking significantly reduced breastmilk production at two weeks postpartum. However, a recent study clearly suggested that nicotine does not alter milk production at all. Therefore, trying to stop smoking by using the nicotine patches is a safer option than continued smoking for breastfeeding mothers. Mothers who choose to use nicotine gum and breastfeed should be counseled to refrain from breastfeeding for several hours after using the gum product. Further, the risk of using nicotine patches while breastfeeding is much less than the risk of formula feeding.

Mothers should be advised to limit smoking as much as possible and to smoke only after they have fed their infant, or to switch to the use of nicotine patches. Under no circumstances should mothers use the patch and smoke simultaneously, as nicotine levels transferred to the infant could be dangerously high.

Relative infant dose:
Time to clear: Between 8 and 10 hours

Lactation risk category: L2
Pregnancy risk category: X if used in overdose
                                            D if used in 3rd trimester
Adult dose: 7-21 milligrams daily
Alternatives:

NICOTINIC ACID

Trade names: Nicobid, Nicolar, Niacels, Niacin,
                            Nicotinamide

AAP recommendation: Not reviewed

Nicotinic acid is commonly called niacin and is converted to nicotinamide in the body. Using high doses may significantly increase the amount present in the mothers' milk, so do not use high doses while breastfeeding. Because niacin is known to be toxic to the liver in higher doses (1-2 grams per day), breastfeeding mothers should not significantly exceed the recommended daily allowance (15 milligrams per day) for niacin unless directed by a physician.

Relative infant dose:
Time to clear: Between 3 and 4 hours
Lactation risk category: L3
Pregnancy risk category: A during 1st and 2nd trimester
                                            C during 3rd trimester
Adult dose: 10-20 milligrams daily
Alternatives:

NIFEDIPINE

Trade names: Adalat, Procardia, Apo-Nifed, Novo-Nifedin,
                            Nu-Nifed, Nifecard, Nyefax, Nefensar XL

AAP recommendation: Maternal medication usually compatible with
                                        breastfeeding

Nifedipine is used in the management of high blood pressure. Nifedipine is transferred into breastmilk in varying, but generally low levels. In two studies, the authors concluded that the amount ingested by the infant via breastmilk posed little risk to the infant. Nifedipine has been found to be clinically useful for nipple vasospasm (blood vessel contraction).

Relative infant dose: 1.9%

Time to clear: Between 7 hours and 1.5 days
Lactation risk category: L2
Pregnancy risk category: C
Adult dose: 10-20 milligrams three times daily
Alternatives: Nimodipine

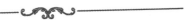

NIMODIPINE

Trade names: Nimotop, Nemotop

AAP recommendation: Not reviewed

Nimodipine is a calcium channel blocker usually given following hemorrhage, acute stroke, and severe head trauma. It is also used to treat migraine headaches. Nimodipine has been reported to be transferred into breastmilk. In two studies, the amount of nimodipine in milk was low. In one study, the authors suggest an infant would ingest approximately 0.008 to 0.092% of the dose administered to the mother.

Relative infant dose: 0.04%
Time to clear: Between 1.5 and 2 days
Lactation risk category: L2
Pregnancy risk category: C
Adult dose: 60 milligrams every 4 hours
Alternatives: Verapamil, Nifedipine.

NISOLDIPINE

Trade names: Sular, Syscor

AAP recommendation: Not reviewed

Nisoldipine is used to treat high blood pressure. There are no reports on the transfer of nisoldipine into breastmilk. However, when considering its chemical properties, it is likely to transfer into breastmilk. For alternatives see nifedipine and verapamil.

Relative infant dose:
Time to clear: Between 1 and 2.5 days
Lactation risk category: L3
Pregnancy risk category: C
Adult dose: 20-40 milligrams daily

Alternatives: Nifedipine, Verapamil, Nimodipine

NITRAZEPAM

Trade names: Mogadon, Nitrazadon, Alodorm, Atempol,
Magadon, Nitrodos

AAP recommendation: Not reviewed

Nitrazepam is used as a sedative. Nitrazepam has been documented to transfer into breastmilk, but no harmful effects were noted in the infants breastfed for 5 days. Nitrazepam levels in a 6 day old infant were not detectable.

Relative infant dose: 2.7%
Time to clear: Between 5 and 6 days
Lactation risk category: L2 (short term)
Pregnancy risk category:
Adult dose: 5-10 milligrams daily
Alternatives: Alprazolam, Lorazepam

NITRENDIPINE

Trade names: Baypress

AAP recommendation: Not reviewed

Nitrendipine is used to treat high blood pressure. It is transferred into breastmilk at low levels. A breastfeeding infant would ingest a very small amount of nitrendipine via breastfeeding. Based on a maternal dose of 20 milligrams daily, a newborn infant would ingest only 0.1% of the maternal dose.

Relative infant dose: 0.1%
Time to clear: Between 1 and 2.5 days
Lactation risk category: L2
Pregnancy risk category:
Adult dose: 10-80 milligrams per day
Alternatives: Nifedipine, Nimodipine

NITROFURANTOIN

Trade names: Furadantin, Macrodantin, Furan, Macrobid,
                   Macrodantin, Nephronex

AAP recommendation: Maternal medication usually compatible with
                          breastfeeding

Nitrofurantoin is an antibiotic that is transferred into breastmilk in very small amounts.   Use with caution in infants with glucose-6-phosphate dehydrogenase deficiency (G6PD) or in infants less than 1 month of age with elevated bilirubin levels. According to the authors, the estimated dose an infant would ingest is only 6.8% of the maternal dose.

Relative infant dose: 6.8%
Time to clear: Between 1.5 and 5 hours
Lactation risk category: L2
Pregnancy risk category: B
Adult dose: 50-100 milligrams four times daily
Alternatives:

NITROGLYCERIN, NITRATES, NITRITES

Trade names: Nitrostat, Nitrolingual, Nitrogard, Imdur,
                   Nitrong, Nitro-Bid, Nitroglyn, Minitran, Nitro-Dur, Nitrol,
                   Anginine, Transderm-Nitro, Isosorbide dinitrate, Nitradisc,
                   Nitrolingual Spray, Deponit

AAP recommendation: Not reviewed

Nitroglycerin, nitrates and nitrites are chemically similar and act about the same way in the body.   Nitroglycerin is used to treat angina and other cardiovascular problems including congestive heart failure. Numerous cases of nitrate toxicity have been reported in infants exposed to well water with high levels of nitrates when they were fed foods/formulas prepared with contaminated water.   It is not clear if nitrates taken orally by the mother transfer into breastmilk in clinically relevant amounts.

Two studies suggest that while nitrates/nitrites are well absorbed orally by the mother (about 50%), little seems to be transferred into breastmilk. While breastmilk levels are not high following the ingestion of oral nitrates, infants younger than 6 months are most at risk for nitrate intoxication.   Breastfeed with caution at higher doses and with prolonged exposure.   Observe the infant for methemoglobinemia.   Isosorbide dinitrate (Imdur, Isordil, etc) are prolonged-released formulations of an organic nitrate vasodilator.   Its transfer into human milk is unknown.

Relative infant dose:
Time to clear: Between 4 and 20 minutes
Lactation risk category: L4
Pregnancy risk category: C
Adult dose: 1.3-6.5 milligrams twice daily

Alternatives:

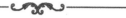

NITROUS OXIDE

Trade names: Entonox
AAP recommendation: Not reviewed

Nitrous oxide is a weak anesthetic gas. It is rapidly removed from the body.
Only tiny traces of nitrous oxide circulate in the blood after gas inhalation
has ended. There are no reports on the entry of nitrous oxide into breastmilk.
Ingestion of nitrous oxide from breastmilk is unlikely. Chronic exposure to
nitrous oxide may lead to elevated risks of fetal malformations, abortions,
and bone marrow toxicity (particular in dental care workers). Waiting to
breastfeed for 30 to 60 minutes following exposure will eliminate any hazard
to the infant.

Relative infant dose:
Time to clear: Between 12 and 15 minutes
Lactation risk category: L3
Pregnancy risk category:
Adult dose: Inhalation 30% with 70% oxygen
Alternatives:

NIZATIDINE

Trade names: Axid, Apo-Nizatidine, Tazac
AAP recommendation: Not reviewed

Nizatidine reduces stomach acid secretion and is used to treat gastric
ulcers, among other uses. Nizatidine is transferred into breastmilk in very
low amounts (less than 0.1% of dose). No effects on infants have been
reported.

Relative infant dose:
Time to clear: Between 6 and 7.5 hours
Lactation risk category: L2

Pregnancy risk category: C
Adult dose: 150-300 milligrams daily
Alternatives: Famotidine

NORELGESTROMIN AND ETHINYL ESTRADIOL

Trade names: Ortho Evra
AAP recommendation: Not reviewed

Ortho Evra is a new combination progestin and estrogen-containing patch. Small amounts of estrogens and progestins are known to pass into breastmilk, although they apparently do not affect the infant. Long-term follow-up of children whose mothers used combination hormonal contraceptives while breastfeeding has shown no harmful effects on infants. Estrogen-containing contraceptives may interfere with milk production by decreasing the quantity and quality of milk production, so we do not advise use of estrogen-containing birth control products.

Relative infant dose:
Time to clear:
Lactation risk category: L3
Pregnancy risk category:
Adult dose: Applied for 7 days times 3 per month.
Alternatives: Norethindrone

NORETHINDRONE

Trade names: Aygestin, Norlutate, Micronor,
NOR-Q.D., Norethisterone, Brevinor
AAP recommendation: Not reviewed

Norethindrone is a typical synthetic progestin used for oral contraception, among other uses. It is believed to be transferred into breastmilk in small amounts. It may decrease the volume of breastmilk to some degree in some mothers if therapy is started too soon after birth (several days) and if the dose is too high. Low dose progestin-only mini pills are the preferred oral contraceptives for breastfeeding mothers.

Relative infant dose:
Time to clear: Between 16 hours and 3 days
Lactation risk category: L1
Pregnancy risk category: X

Adult dose: 0.35-5 milligrams daily
Alternatives:

NORETHYNODREL

Trade names: Enovid
AAP recommendation: Maternal medication usually compatible with
                        breastfeeding

Norethynodrel is a synthetic progestin used in oral contraceptives. It has
limited or no effects on the infant. It may decrease the volume of breastmilk
to some degree in some mothers if therapy is initiated too soon after birth (2
days) and if the dose is too high. See norethindrone, medroxyprogesterone.

Relative infant dose:
Time to clear:
Lactation risk category: L2
Pregnancy risk category: X
Adult dose:
Alternatives:

NORFLOXACIN

Trade names: Noroxin
AAP recommendation: Not reviewed

Norfloxacin is a member of the fluoroquinolone antibiotic family. Although
other members in this antibiotic family are secreted into breastmilk (see
ciprofloxacin, ofloxacin), there are only limited reports on the transfer of
norfloxacin in breastmilk. One author suggested that norfloxacin is not
present in breastmilk. The manufacturer's product information states that
doses of 200 milligrams do not produce detectable amounts in milk; although,
this was a single dose. Norfloxacin, levofloxacin, or perhaps ofloxacin may
be preferred for use in breastfeeding mothers.

Relative infant dose:
Time to clear: Between 13 and 16.5 hours
Lactation risk category: L3
Pregnancy risk category: C
Adult dose: 400 milligrams twice daily
Alternatives: Ofloxacin, Levofloxacin

NORTRIPTYLINE

Trade names: Aventyl, Pamelor, Norventyl, Allegron,
                 Apo-Nortriptyline

AAP recommendation: Drug whose effect on nursing infants is
                        unknown but may be of concern

Nortriptyline is an antidepressant and is the active metabolite of amitriptyline (Elavil). Although one study found nortriptyline in breastmilk, several other authors have been unable to detect it in breastmilk or in the blood of infants after prolonged exposure. So far, no harmful effects have been noted.

Relative infant dose: 1.5%
Time to clear: Between 2.5 and 19 days
Lactation risk category: L2
Pregnancy risk category: D
Adult dose: 25 milligrams three to four times daily
Alternatives: Imipramine

NYSTATIN

Trade names: Mycostatin, Nilstat, Nadostine, Candistatin,
                 Nystan

AAP recommendation: Not reviewed

Nystatin is an antifungal primarily used to treat candidiasis topically (applied on the skin) and thrush in the infant's mouth. The oral absorption of nystatin is extremely poor and blood levels are undetectable after taken orally. The likelihood of the transfer of nystatin into breastmilk is remote due to poor maternal absorption. It is frequently given to neonates in neonatal units for candidiasis. In addition, absorption into the infant's blood is equally unlikely.

Relative infant dose:
Time to clear:
Lactation risk category: L1
Pregnancy risk category: B
Adult dose: 500,000-1 million units three times daily
Alternatives: Fluconazole

OFLOXACIN

Trade names: Floxin, Ocuflox, Tarivid

AAP recommendation: Maternal medication usually compatible with breastfeeding

Ofloxacin is an antibiotic that belongs to the fluoroquinolone family of drugs. Breastmilk concentrations are reported equal to maternal plasma levels. Ofloxacin was still found in breastmilk 24 hours after a maternal dose. The fluoroquinolones are becoming more popular in pediatrics due to recent studies and reviews showing their safe use. The only probable risk is a change in gut flora, diarrhea, and a remote risk of severe diarrhea. Ofloxacin levels in breastmilk are consistently lower (37%) than ciprofloxacin. If a fluoroquinolone is required, ofloxacin, levofloxacin, or norfloxacin are probably the preferred choices for breastfeeding mothers.

Relative infant dose: < 3.1%
Time to clear: Between 20 and 35 hours
Lactation risk category: L2
Pregnancy risk category: C
Adult dose: 200-400 milligrams twice daily
Alternatives: Norfloxacin, Levofloxacin

OLANZAPINE

Trade names: Zyprexa, Symbyax

AAP recommendation: Not reviewed

Olanzapine is a typical antipsychotic agent structurally similar to clozapine and is used to treat psychosis. In one study, olanzapine was not detected in the plasma of six infants tested. All infants were healthy and had no observable side effects. In another case, no levels were reported in breastmilk and no effects were noted in the infant. The new product, Symbyax, contains both fluoxetine and olanzapine and is used to treat Bipolar Depression.

Relative infant dose: 1.2%
Time to clear: Between 3.5 and 11.5 days
Lactation risk category: L2
Pregnancy risk category: C
Adult dose: 5-10 milligrams daily
Alternatives: Risperidone, Haloperidol

OLMESARTAN MEDOXOMIL

Trade names: Benicar, Benicar HCT

AAP recommendation: Not reviewed

Olmesartan (Benicar) and olmesartan plus a diuretic - hydrochlorothiazide (Benicar HCT) are used in the management of high blood pressure. Use in pregnancy is contraindicated. There are no reports on the transfer of olmesartan into breastmilk, but its use in newborn infants could be risky.

Relative infant dose:
Time to clear: Between 2 and 3 days
Lactation risk category: L3 in older infants
Pregnancy risk category: C in 1st trimester
D in 2nd and 3rd trimester
Adult dose: 20-40 milligrams daily
Alternatives: Captopril, Enalapril

OLOPATADINE OPHTHALMIC

Trade names: Patanol, Opatanol

AAP recommendation: Not reviewed

Olopatadine is an antihistamine used in the treatment of allergic conjunctivitis. It is used topically in the eye. The manufacturer suggest that absorption is low in adults and that plasma levels are undetectable in most cases. Because adult plasma levels are so low, it is very unlikely any would be detectable in breastmilk. However, there are no reports on the levels in breastmilk, but the risk is probably quite low.

Relative infant dose:
Time to clear: Between 12 and 15 hours
Lactation risk category: L2
Pregnancy risk category: C
Adult dose: One drop in affected eye twice daily.
Alternatives:

OLSALAZINE

Trade names: Dipentum

AAP recommendation: Not reviewed

Olsalazine is converted to 5-aminosalicylic acid in the gut and produces an anti-inflammatory activity in ulcerative colitis. After being taken orally, only 2.4% is absorbed while the majority is broken down in the gastrointestinal tract to 5-aminosalicylic acid. 5-Aminosalicylic acid is slowly and poorly absorbed with exceedingly small blood levels. While clinically significant levels in breastmilk are unlikely, infants should be closely monitored for gastric changes such as watery diarrhea.

Relative infant dose: 0.9%
Time to clear: Between 3.5 and 4.5 hours
Lactation risk category: L3
Pregnancy risk category: C
Adult dose: 500 milligrams twice daily
Alternatives:

OMEPRAZOLE

Trade names: Prilosec, Losec

AAP recommendation: Not reviewed

Omeprazole is used to treat stomach acidity and duodenal ulcers. The amount of omeprazole in breastmilk is very low. Most, if not all, of the omeprazole ingested via breastmilk would be destroyed in the stomach of the infant prior to absorption.

Relative infant dose:
Time to clear: Between 4 and 5 hours
Lactation risk category: L2
Pregnancy risk category: C
Adult dose: 20 milligrams twice daily
Alternatives: Famotidine, Nizatidine

ONDANSETRON

Trade names: Zofran

AAP recommendation: Not reviewed

Ondansetron is used clinically to reduce nausea and vomiting linked to chemotherapy. It has occasionally been used during pregnancy without effect on the fetus. It is available for oral and intravenous administration. There are no reports on the transfer of ondansetron into breastmilk, but it is probably safe.

Relative infant dose:
Time to clear: Between 14.5 and 18 hours
Lactation risk category: L2
Pregnancy risk category: B
Adult dose: 8 milligrams twice daily
Alternatives:

ORAL CONTRACEPTIVES

Trade names: Norinyl, Norlestin, Ovral, Ortho-Novum,
                Nornyl, Cilest, Brevinor

AAP recommendation: Maternal medication usually compatible with
                      breastfeeding

Oral contraceptives, particularly those containing estrogens, tend to reduce lactose production, reducing the volume of milk produced. Quality (fat content) may similarly be reduced; although, one recent study of the fat, energy, protein, and lactose concentration in milk of mothers using oral contraceptives showed no effect from the contraceptives. The earlier the oral contraceptives are started, the greater the negative effect on lactation.

Although it was previously believed that waiting 6 weeks would prevent breastfeeding problems, this is apparently not accurate. Numerous examples of milk supply problems have occurred after the first six weeks in some patients. It is suggested that the mother establish a good milk flow (60-90 days) before starting oral contraceptives. Use progestin-only mini pills or, if necessary, use only LOW DOSE combination oral contraceptives with 35-50 mcg of estrogen.

Alternates, such as progestin-only oral contraceptives (rather than Depo-Provera), are suggested so that if a supply problems occur the patient can easily withdraw from the medication. Depo-Provera should only be used in those patients who have used it previously and have not experienced breastmilk supply problems or in those who have used progestin-only mini pills without problems. Try to wait 6 weeks postpartum before using Depo-Provera. The progestins and estrogens present in breastmilk (from the oral contraceptives) are quite low and numerous studies confirm that they have minimal or no effect on sexual development in infants.

Relative infant dose:
Time to clear:
Lactation risk category: L3
Pregnancy risk category: X
Adult dose:
Alternatives: Norethindrone

ORPHENADRINE CITRATE

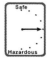

Trade names: Norflex, Banflex, Norgesic, Myotrol,
                  Orfenace, Disipal
AAP recommendation: Not reviewed

Orphenadrine is related to Benadryl. It is primarily used as a muscle relaxant. There are no reports on the transfer of orphenadrine into breastmilk.

Relative infant dose:
Time to clear: Between 2.5 and 3 days
Lactation risk category: L3
Pregnancy risk category: C
Adult dose: 100 milligrams twice daily
Alternatives:

OSELTAMIVIR PHOSPHATE

Trade names: Tamiflu
AAP recommendation: Not reviewed

Tamiflu is used to treat uncomplicated acute illness due to influenza A and B infection in adults who have had symptoms for no more than 2 days. Tamiflu is only moderately effective. About 75% is available to the body following oral administration. It is not known if Tamiflu transfers into breastmilk, but the levels would likely be incredibly low due to the low maternal plasma levels. However, due to its limited effectiveness, its use in breastfeeding mothers is probably not warranted, unless in high-risk patients with other severe medical conditions.

Relative infant dose:
Time to clear: Between 1 and 2 days
Lactation risk category: L3
Pregnancy risk category: C
Adult dose: 75 milligrams twice daily for 5 days.
Alternatives:

OSMOTIC LAXATIVES

Trade names: Milk of Magnesia, Fleet Phospho-Soda,
Citrate of Magnesia, Epsom salt, Citromag, Sorbilax,
Duphalac

AAP recommendation: Not reviewed

Osmotic or Saline laxatives are comprised of a large number of magnesium and phosphate compounds, but all work by pulling and retaining water into the gastrointestinal tract, thus functioning as laxatives. Because they are poorly absorbed, they primarily stay in the gastrointestinal tract and are eliminated without significant systemic absorption. The small amount of magnesium and phosphate salts absorbed are rapidly cleared by the kidneys. Products considered osmotic laxatives include: Milk of Magnesia, Epsom Salts, Citrate of Magnesia, Fleets Phospho-soda, and other sodium phosphate compounds.

Relative infant dose:
Time to clear:
Lactation risk category: L1
Pregnancy risk category: C
Adult dose:
Alternatives:

OXAPROZIN

Trade names: Daypro

AAP recommendation: Not reviewed

Oxaprozin belongs to the non-steroidal anti-inflammatory drug (NSAID) family of pain killers. It is reported to have lesser gastrointestinal side effects than certain other NSAIDs. There are no reports on the transfer of oxaprozin into breastmilk. Although its long half-life could cause problems in breastfed infants, it is probably poorly transferred to human milk.

Relative infant dose:
Time to clear: Between 7 and 10.5 days
Lactation risk category: L3
Pregnancy risk category: C
Adult dose: 600-1200 milligrams daily
Alternatives: Ibuprofen, Celecoxib

OXAZEPAM

Trade names: Serax, Novoxapam, Zapex, Alepam,
                            Murelax, Serepax, Oxanid
AAP recommendation: Not reviewed

Oxazepam belongs to the benzodiazepine family of drugs (see valium) and is used in anxiety disorders. Of the benzodiazepines, oxazepam is the least lipid soluble. In one reported patient, milk levels were exceedingly low.

Relative infant dose: 1.1%
Time to clear: Between 2 and 2.5 days
Lactation risk category: L3
Pregnancy risk category: D
Adult dose: 10-30 milligrams three to four times daily
Alternatives:

OXCARBAZEPINE

Trade names: Trileptal
AAP recommendation: Not reviewed

Oxcarbazepine is derived from carbamazepine (Tegretol) and is used to treat seizures in adults and children. The transfer of oxycarbazepine into milk is reportedly low and tends to fall significantly (93%) in the 5 days following delivery of the drug.

Relative infant dose:
Time to clear: Between 1.5 and 2 days
Lactation risk category: L3
Pregnancy risk category: C
Adult dose: 300-600 milligrams twice daily
Alternatives: Carbamazepine

OXYBUTYNIN

Trade names: Ditropan, Apo-Oxybutynin, Oxybutyn

AAP recommendation: Not reviewed

Oxybutynin is an antispasmodic used for conditions with symptoms of involuntary bladder spasms. It reduces urinary urgency and frequency. There are no reports on the transfer of this drug into breastmilk. Oxybutynin has a chemical structure which is unlikely to be transferred into breastmilk. While milk levels are unreported, they are almost certainly low and clinically irrelevant to even a neonate.

Relative infant dose:
Time to clear: Between 4 and 10 hours
Lactation risk category: L3
Pregnancy risk category: B
Adult dose: 5 milligrams two to four times daily
Alternatives:

OXYCODONE

Trade names: Tylox, Percodan, OxyContin, Roxicet,
Endocet, Roxiprin, Percocet, Endone, Proladone

AAP recommendation: Not reviewed

Oxycodone is similar to hydrocodone and is a potent pain killer significantly stronger than codeine. Small to moderate amounts are secreted into breastmilk. No reports of harmful effects in infants have been found; although, sedation is a possibility in some infants. Endocet, Percocet, Roxicet and Roxiprin are all formulations of oxycodone and acetaminophen. Use this drug sparingly, spacing doses so as to not sedate your infant.

Relative infant dose: 4.0%
Time to clear: Between 12 and 30 hours
Lactation risk category: L3
Pregnancy risk category: B
Adult dose: 5 milligrams every 6 hours
Alternatives: Codeine

OXYTOCIN

Trade names: Pitocin, Syntocinon, Syntometrine

AAP recommendation: Not reviewed

Oxytocin is produced by the pituitary gland and is responsible for the let-down response that forces milk from the breast. Oxytocin is available as injections for intravenous and intranasal use. If it is taken orally, it is instantly destroyed. The oral absorption in neonates is unknown but probably minimal. No harmful effects have been noted in breastfeeding infants. Oxytocin is sometimes used intranasally in rare cases to cause let-down. Chronic use of intranasal oxytocin may lead to dependence and should be limited to the first week postpartum.

Relative infant dose:
Time to clear: Between 12 and 25 minutes
Lactation risk category: L2
Pregnancy risk category:
Adult dose: 40-80 units daily
Alternatives:

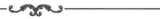

PACLITAXEL

Trade names: Taxol, Anzatax

AAP recommendation: Not reviewed

Paclitaxel is a plant product that is used in the management of cancer. It is derived from the bark of the western yew tree. Structurally paclitaxel is a large chemical which reduces its ability to enter milk. It is not known if paclitaxel enters breastmilk, but due to the extraordinary toxicity and lipid solubility of this compound, it would not be advisable to breastfeed while using this drug.

Relative infant dose:
Time to clear: Between 2 and 11 days
Lactation risk category: L5
Pregnancy risk category: D
Adult dose: 135-175 milligrams per meter squared every 3 weeks
Alternatives:

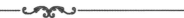

PAMIDRONATE

Trade names: Aredia

AAP recommendation: Not reviewed

Pamidronate inhibits bone-reabsorption. One study was performed on a woman who received pamidronate through intravenous injections once a month. None was found in her breastmilk. The authors suggested that pamidronate could be considered safe for use in lactating women. Pamidronate is poorly absorbed orally (0.3% to 3% of a dose) and it is unlikely any would be absorbed by the infant from breastmilk.

Relative infant dose:
Time to clear: Between 4.5 and 6 days
Lactation risk category: L2
Pregnancy risk category: C
Adult dose: 60 to 90 milligrams as a single intravenous drip
Alternatives:

PANTOPRAZOLE

Trade names: Protonix

AAP recommendation: Not reviewed

Pantoprazole belongs to the family of drugs called the proton-pump inhibitors. Pantoprazole is similar to omeprazole (Prilosec) and is used in the treatment of reflux and gastric ulcers. The manufacturer reports 0.02% of an administered dose is transferred into breastmilk. As with all the proton-pump inhibitors, pantoprazole is unstable in an acid environment (stomach). When present in breastmilk, it would be broken down in the infant's stomach and not absorbed. See omeprazole for an alternative.

Relative infant dose:
Time to clear: Between 4 and 5 hours
Lactation risk category: L2
Pregnancy risk category: B
Adult dose: 40-80 milligrams daily
Alternatives: Omeprazole

PAREGORIC

Trade names:

AAP recommendation: Not reviewed

Paregoric is camphorated tincture of opium. It contains approximately 2 milligrams of morphine per teaspoonful in 45% alcohol. Because the active ingredient is morphine, see morphine for breastfeeding indications. Due to its camphor content, the use of paregoric in infants and children is discouraged.

Relative infant dose:
Time to clear: Between 6 and 10 hours
Lactation risk category: L3
Pregnancy risk category: B
Adult dose: 5-10 milliliters (2-4 milligrams morphine) two to four
                   times daily
Alternatives:

PAROXETINE

Trade names: Paxil, Aropax 20, Seroxat

AAP recommendation: Drug whose effect on nursing infants is
                         unknown but may be of concern

Paroxetine is used to treat depression. Almost 60 breastfeeding mother/infants have been studied and all studies conclude that the amount of paroxetine transferred into breastmilk is minimal. Based on studies performed, paroxetine can be considered relatively 'safe' for use in breastfeeding mothers.

Relative infant dose: 2.1%
Time to clear: Between 3.5 and 4.5 days
Lactation risk category: L2
Pregnancy risk category: B
Adult dose: 20-50 milligrams daily
Alternatives: Sertraline

PEMOLINE

Trade names: Cylert, Kethamed, Ronyl

AAP recommendation: Not reviewed

Pemoline is used to treat attention deficit/hyperactivity disorder (ADHD) and is very similar to amphetamine and Ritalin (methylphenidate). At present, there are no reports on the transfer of pemoline into breastmilk, but it is likely due to its low molecular weight. Maternal peak level occurs 2-4 hrs after dose. It was recently removed from the US market.

Relative infant dose:
Time to clear: Between 2 and 2.5 days
Lactation risk category: L4
Pregnancy risk category: C
Adult dose: 50-200 milligrams daily
Alternatives:

PENCICLOVIR

Trade names: Denavir, Vectavir

AAP recommendation: Not reviewed

Penciclovir is an antiviral agent used to treat cold sores (herpes simplex) of the lips and face and occasionally for herpes zoster (Shingles). Following topical administration, plasma levels are undetectable. Because maternal plasma levels are undetectable following topical therapy, it is extremely unlikely that detectable amounts would transfer into breastmilk or be absorbed by an infant.

Relative infant dose:
Time to clear: Between 9 and 11.5 hours
Lactation risk category: L3
Pregnancy risk category: B
Adult dose: Topical application every 2 hours
Alternatives:

PENICILLAMINE

Trade names: Cuprimine, Depen, D-Penamine, Distamine, Pendramine

AAP recommendation: Not reviewed

Penicillamine is a potent binding agent used to treat high blood levels of copper, iron, mercury, lead, and other metals. It is also used to suppress the immune response in rheumatoid arthritis and other such syndromes. It is extremely dangerous during pregnancy. Safety has not been established during lactation. Penicillamine is a potent drug that requires constant observation and care by attending physicians. Discontinuation of lactation is recommended if this drug is mandatory.

Relative infant dose:
Time to clear: Between 7 and 16 hours
Lactation risk category: L4
Pregnancy risk category: D
Adult dose: 250-500 milligrams four times daily
Alternatives:

PENICILLIN G

Trade names: Pfizerpen, Megacillin, Ayercillin, Crystapen, Bicillin L-A

AAP recommendation: Maternal medication usually compatible with breastfeeding

Penicillin G is an antibiotic. Penicillins generally enter breastmilk in small amounts, largely determined by their class. Penicillin G is poorly transferred into breastmilk even following injections into the muscle at doses of 100,000 units. Possible side effects in infants would include changes in gastrointestinal flora or allergic responses in an allergic infant. This drug is compatible with breastfeeding in non-hypersensitive infants.

Relative infant dose:
Time to clear: Between 6 and 7.5 hours
Lactation risk category: L1
Pregnancy risk category: B
Adult dose: 1.2-2.4 million units daily
Alternatives:

PENTOBARBITAL

Trade names: Nembutal, Nova-Rectal, Novo-Pentobarb,
Barbopen, Carbrital, Lethobarb

AAP recommendation: Not reviewed

Pentobarbital belongs to the barbiturate family and is primarily used as a sedative. The effect of short-acting barbiturates on the breastfed infant is unknown, but significant tolerance and addiction can occur. Use caution if used in large amounts.

Relative infant dose: 1.8%
Time to clear: Between 2.5 and 10.5 days
Lactation risk category: L3
Pregnancy risk category: D
Adult dose: 20-40 milligrams two to four times daily
Alternatives:

PENTOSAN POLYSULFATE

Trade names: Elmiron

AAP recommendation: Not reviewed

Pentosan polysulfate is used as a urinary tract analgesic. It is structurally related to dextran sulfate and has a very high molecular weight, thus it would have difficulty entering milk. Although there are no reports on its transfer into breastmilk, its large molecular weight and poor oral absorption would largely prevent the transfer and absorption of clinically relevant amounts into milk and therefore breastfed infants.

Relative infant dose:
Time to clear: Between 20 and 25 hours
Lactation risk category: L2
Pregnancy risk category: B
Adult dose: 100 milligrams three times daily
Alternatives:

PERMETHRIN

Trade names: Nix, Elimite, A-200, Pyrinex, Pyrinyl,
Acticin, Lyclear, Pyrifoam, Quellada

AAP recommendation: Not reviewed

Permethrin is used to treat lice, mites, and fleas. Permethrin absorption through the skin following application of a 5% cream is reported to be less than 2%. Permethrin is rapidly broken down by serum enzymes and rapidly excreted in the urine, so it is quite safe. It is not known if permethrin is secreted into breastmilk. Since this product can be used directly on infants, it should be acceptable for breastfeeding mothers.

Relative infant dose:
Time to clear:
Lactation risk category: L2
Pregnancy risk category: B
Adult dose:
Alternatives:

PERPHENAZINE AND AMITRIPTYLINE

Trade names: Triavil, Etrafon

AAP recommendation: Drug whose effect on nursing infants is unknown but may be of concern

Perphenazine is commonly combined in the USA with amitriptyline. The combination drug is called Etrafon or Triavil. See amitriptyline for more details. Perphenazine is used as an antipsychotic or sedative. It is transferred into breastmilk in moderate levels. The authors of one study reported that during a 3 month exposure, the infant thrived and had no adverse response to the drug. They also estimated the dose to be about 0.1% of the maternal dose.

Relative infant dose: 0.1% (perphenazine)
Time to clear: Between 1 and 2.5 days
Lactation risk category: L3
Pregnancy risk category: C
Adult dose: 12-64 milligrams daily
Alternatives:

PHENAZOPYRIDINE HCL

Trade names: Pyridium, Eridium, Azo-Standard, Pyronium, Uromide

AAP recommendation: Not reviewed

Phenazopyridine (Pyridium) is a dye that is rapidly excreted in the urine where it provides pain relief in the bladder. Pyridium is only moderately effective and colors the urine reddish-orange. It can stain clothing and ruin contact lenses. It is not known if Pyridium transfers into breastmilk, but it probably does to a limited degree. This product, due to limited effectiveness, should probably not be used in lactating women; although, it is doubtful that it would be harmful to an infant.

Relative infant dose:
Time to clear:
Lactation risk category: L3
Pregnancy risk category: B
Adult dose: 100-200 milligrams three times daily
Alternatives:

PHENCYCLIDINE

Common names: PCP, Angel dust

AAP recommendation: Contraindicated by the American Academy of Pediatrics in breastfeeding mothers

Phencyclidine, also called Angel Dust, is a potent and extremely dangerous hallucinogen. It is transferred into breastmilk and may be secreted into breastmilk over long periods of time (perhaps months). PCP IS EXTREMELY DANGEROUS TO NURSING INFANTS. Urine samples are positive for 14-30 days in adults and probably longer in infants. The infant could test positive for PCP long after maternal exposure (many weeks), particularly if breastfeeding. The mother should pump and discard her milk for at least two weeks after use.

Relative infant dose:
Time to clear: Between 4 and 10.5 days
Lactation risk category: L5
Pregnancy risk category: X
Adult dose:
Alternatives:

PHENOBARBITAL

Trade names: Luminal, Phenobarbitone, Gardenal

AAP recommendation: Drug associated with significant side effects and should be taken with caution

Phenobarbital belongs to the barbiturate family of drugs. It is frequently used as an anticonvulsant in adults and neonates. Its long half-life in infants may lead to significant accumulation and blood levels higher than in the mother; although, this is infrequent. The half-life in premature infants can be extremely long (100-500 hours) and plasma levels must be closely monitored. Phenobarbital should be administered with caution and close observation of the infant is required, including measuring drug levels in blood. One should generally expect the infant's plasma level to be approximately 30-40% of the maternal level.

Relative infant dose: 24.0%
Time to clear: Between 9 and 29 days
Lactation risk category: L3
Pregnancy risk category: D
Adult dose: 100-200 milligrams daily
Alternatives:

PHENYLEPHRINE

Trade names: Neo-Synephrine, AK-Dilate, Dionephrine, Vicks Sinex Nasal, Albalone, Fenox

AAP recommendation: Not reviewed

Phenylephrine is most commonly used as a nasal decongestant due to its vasoconstrictive properties. It is also for treatment of ocular uveitis (eye inflammation), glaucoma, and cardiogenic shock. Phenylephrine is most commonly added to cold mixtures and nasal sprays for use in respiratory colds, flu, and congestion. Numerous pediatric formulations are in use and it is generally considered safe in pediatric patients. There are no reports on its secretion into breastmilk, but it is likely that small amounts will probably be transferred. Due to its poor oral bioavailability (< 38%), it is not likely to produce clinical effects in a breastfed infant unless the maternal doses are quite high.

Relative infant dose:
Time to clear: Between 8 and 15 hours
Lactation risk category: L3
Pregnancy risk category: C

Adult dose: 1-10 milligrams injection into the muscle
Alternatives: Pseudoephedrine

PHENYTOIN

Trade names: Dilantin, Novo-Phenytoin, Epanutin

AAP recommendation: Maternal medication usually compatible with
                         breastfeeding

Phenytoin is an old and efficient anticonvulsant that is sometimes used in
infant seizure disorders. All of the current studies indicate rather low levels of
phenytoin in breastmilk and minimal plasma levels in breastfeeding infants.
The effect on the breastfeeding infant is generally considered minimal if
the mother's blood levels are kept in low-normal range (10 micrograms per
milliliters). The neonatal half-life of phenytoin is highly variable for the first
week of life. Monitoring of the infants' plasma may be useful; although, it
is not required.

Relative infant dose: 7.7%
Time to clear: Between 1 and 5 days
Lactation risk category: L2
Pregnancy risk category: D
Adult dose: 300 milligrams daily
Alternatives:

PHYTONADIONE

Trade names: Phytonadione, AquaMephyton, Konakion,
                  Mephyton, Vitamin K1

AAP recommendation: Maternal medication usually compatible with
                         breastfeeding

Phytonadione (Vitamin K1) is often used to reverse the effects of oral
anticoagulants and to prevent hemorrhagic disease of the newborn (HDN,
a bleeding problem in neonates). Although controversial, it is thought that
breastmilk may not have enough vitamin K1 to provide normal clotting
factors, particularly in the premature infant or those with GI absorptive
disorders. Vitamin K concentration in breastmilk is normally low and most
infants are born with low coagulation factors (30-60% of normal). Although
vitamin K is transferred into breastmilk, the amount may not be sufficient to
prevent hemorrhagic disease of the newborn.

Vitamin K requires the presence of bile and other factors for absorption, so neonatal absorption may be slow or delayed. A single injection into the muscle of the infant of 0.5 to 1 milligram or an oral dose of 1-2 milligrams during the neonatal period is recommended by the AAP. Use of Vitamin K in breastfeeding mothers is safe.

Relative infant dose:
Time to clear:
Lactation risk category: L1
Pregnancy risk category: C
Adult dose: 65 micrograms daily
Alternatives:

PILOCARPINE

Trade names: Isopto Carpine, Pilocar, Akarpine,
                   Ocusert Pilo

AAP recommendation: Not reviewed

Pilocarpine is used primarily in the eyes for treatment of glaucoma. It is not known if pilocarpine enters breastmilk, but it probably does in low levels. It is not likely that an infant would receive a clinical dose via breastmilk, but this is presently unknown. Side effects include diarrhea, gastric upset and excessive salivation.

Relative infant dose:
Time to clear: Between 3 and 8 hours
Lactation risk category: L3
Pregnancy risk category: C
Adult dose: 5-10 milligrams three times daily
Alternatives:

PIMECROLIMUS

Trade names: Elidel

AAP recommendation: Not reviewed

Pimecrolimus is a topical agent used for atopic dermatitis (allergic reaction and inflammation of the skin). Systemic absorption following topical application is minimal. There are no reports on its transfer into breastmilk. Because the maternal plasma levels are so low, it is very unlikely that pimecrolimus would penetrate breastmilk in clinically relevant amounts.

However, its use on or around the nipples should be avoided as the clinical dose absorbed orally by the infant could be significant.

Relative infant dose:
Time to clear:
Lactation risk category: L2
                                              L4 on nipple
Pregnancy risk category: C
Adult dose: Apply twice daily to skin.
Alternatives:

PIMOZIDE

Trade names: Orap
AAP recommendation: Not reviewed

Pimozide is a potent drug primarily used for Tourette's syndrome and chronic schizophrenia. Pimozide induces a low degree of sedation. There are no reports on the transfer of pimozide into breastmilk. The benefit to the mother must be weighed against the possible danger to the child. Extreme caution is suggested.

Relative infant dose:
Time to clear: Between 9 and 11.5 days
Lactation risk category: L4
Pregnancy risk category: C
Adult dose: 7-16 milligrams daily
Alternatives:

PIOGLITAZONE

Trade names: Actos
AAP recommendation: Not reviewed

Pioglitazone is used in the management of non-insulin dependent diabetes mellitus (Type 2). There are no reports on the transfer of pioglitazone into breastmilk. See metformin as an alternative.

Relative infant dose:
Time to clear: Between 2.5 and 5 days
Lactation risk category: L3
Pregnancy risk category: C
Adult dose: 15-30 milligrams once daily

Alternatives: Metformin

PIPERACILLIN

Trade names: Zosyn, Pipracil, Pipril, Tazocin

AAP recommendation: Not reviewed

Piperacillin is a penicillin antibiotic that is not absorbed orally. When combined with tazobactam sodium, it is called Zosyn. The amount of piperacillin transferred into breastmilk is believed to be extremely low. Its poor oral absorption would limit its absorption in the infant.

Relative infant dose:
Time to clear: Between 2.5 and 6.5 hours
Lactation risk category: L2
Pregnancy risk category: B
Adult dose: 4-5 grams two to three times daily
Alternatives:

PIRBUTEROL ACETATE

Trade names: Maxair, Evirel

AAP recommendation: Not reviewed

Pirbuterol is used to treat asthma. The inhaler form is more common, but the oral form is occasionally prescribed. There are no reports on the levels of pirbuterol in breastmilk. The amount absorbed in the mother would probably be minimal following the use of the inhaler. If using the the oral formulation, the amount in the plasma would be much higher and would be associated with a higher risk for breastfeeding infants.

Relative infant dose:
Time to clear: Between 8 and 15 hours
Lactation risk category: L2
Pregnancy risk category: C
Adult dose: 0.2-0.4 milligrams every 4-6 hours
Alternatives:

PIROXICAM

Trade names: Feldene, Novo-Pirocam, Candyl, Mobilis, Pirox

AAP recommendation: Maternal medication usually compatible with breastfeeding

Piroxicam is a typical non-steroidal anti-inflammatory drug (NSAID) commonly used to treat arthritis. Even though piroxicam has a very long half-life, one report suggests its use to be safe in breastfeeding mothers. The daily dose ingested by the infant was calculated to average 3.5% of the maternal dose.

Relative infant dose: 4.1%
Time to clear: Between 5 and 18 days
Lactation risk category: L2
Pregnancy risk category: B
Adult dose: 20 milligrams daily
Alternatives: Ibuprofen

POLYETHYLENE GLYCOL-ELECTROLYTE SOLUTIONS

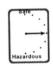

Trade names: GoLYTELY, Col-Lav, Colovage, CoLyte, OCL

AAP recommendation: Not reviewed

Polyethylene glycol-electrolyte solution (PEG-ES) is a saline laxative. It is a non-absorbable solution used to cleanse the bowel prior to surgical procedures and colonoscopy. It is completely unabsorbed from the adult gastrointestinal tract and is unlikely to penetrate breastmilk. This product is often used in children and infants prior to gastrointestinal surgery. Although there are no reports on the transfer of PEG-ES into breastmilk, it is very unlikely that enough maternal absorption would occur to produce significant levels of PEG-ES in breastmilk.

Relative infant dose:
Time to clear:
Lactation risk category: L3
Pregnancy risk category: C
Adult dose: 240 milliliters every 10 minutes up to 4 liters
Alternatives:

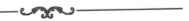

POTASSIUM IODIDE

Trade names: SSKI

AAP recommendation: Not reviewed

Potassium iodide is often used to suppress thyroxine secretion in hyperthyroid (overactive thyroid gland) patients. It is also used to prevent the absorption of radioactive iodine following exposure to this radioisotope. Iodide salts are known to be secreted into breastmilk in high concentrations. Iodides are captured in the thyroid gland at high levels and can potentially cause severe thyroid depression in a breastfed infant. Use with extreme caution if at all.

Relative infant dose:
Time to clear:
Lactation risk category: L4
Pregnancy risk category: D
Adult dose: 5-10 milligrams daily
Alternatives:

POVIDONE IODIDE

Trade names: Betadine, Iodex, Operand, Pharmadine,
                  Proviodine, Isodine, Viodine, Minidine

AAP recommendation: Maternal medication usually compatible with
                         breastfeeding

Povidone iodide is mainly used as an antiseptic and antimicrobial. Very little iodide is absorbed when applied to the skin. Significant and increased plasma levels of iodine have been documented when used as a douche (povidone-iodine douche). The topical application to infants has resulted in significant absorption through the skin. Once plasma levels are attained in the mother, iodide rapidly transfers into breastmilk in high levels. See potassium iodide. High oral iodine intake, and even the use of povidone douches in mothers is documented to produce thyroid suppression in breastfed infants. Use with extreme caution or not at all. Repeated use of povidone iodide is not recommended in nursing mothers or their infants.

Relative infant dose:
Time to clear:
Lactation risk category: L4
Pregnancy risk category: D
Adult dose:

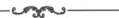

Alternatives:

PRAZEPAM

Trade names: Centrax

AAP recommendation: Drug whose effect on nursing infants is unknown but may be of concern

Prazepam is part of the "Valium" sedative family of drugs. There are no reports on the transfer of prazepam into breastmilk. Most benzodiazepines readily transfer into milk, though most levels are not clinically relevant. Observe the infant closely for sedation. See diazepam.

Relative infant dose:
Time to clear: Between 5 and 21 days
Lactation risk category: L3
Pregnancy risk category: D
Adult dose: 10 milligrams three times daily
Alternatives: Lorazepam, Alprazolam

PREDNISONE - PREDNISOLONE

Trade names: Prednisone, Prednisolone

AAP recommendation: Maternal medication usually compatible with breastfeeding

Prednisone and prednisolone are steroids used to reduce inflammation. Only small amounts (0.14%) of most corticosteroids are transferred into breastmilk. Even in larger doses (100 milligrams per day) these two steroids are not contraindicated in nursing mothers. The steroids used in asthmatics (inhaled) are definitely not contraindicated and mothers can safely breastfeed. When using high doses for longer periods, steroids can potentially cause problems although none have been reported. Brief applications of high dose steroids are probably not contraindicated as the overall exposure is low.

Relative infant dose: 2.0%
Time to clear: Between 4 and 5 days
Lactation risk category: L2
Pregnancy risk category: C
Adult dose: 5-120 milligrams per day
Alternatives:

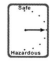

PROCAINE HCL

Trade names: Novocaine

AAP recommendation: Not reviewed

Procaine is a local anesthetic with low potential for systemic toxicity and short duration of action. Procaine is rapidly metabolized. There are no reports on the transfer of procaine into breastmilk, but it is unlikely. Most other local anesthetics (see bupivacaine, lidocaine) transfer into breastmilk in small amounts. It is likely that procaine, due to its brief plasma half-life, would produce even lower milk levels. When considering its chemical properties, any amount transferred would be poorly absorbed by the infant.

Relative infant dose:
Time to clear: Between 31 and 38.5 minutes
Lactation risk category: L3
Pregnancy risk category: C
Adult dose: 350-600 milligrams once
Alternatives:

PROCHLORPERAZINE

Trade names: Compazine, Stemetil, Nu-Prochlor,
                 Buccastem

AAP recommendation: Not reviewed

Prochlorperazine is used as a sedataive and to treat nausea/vomiting. There are no reports on the levels of prochlorperazine in breastmilk, but other similar drugs enter breastmilk in small amounts. Because infants are extremely hypersensitive to these compounds, caution is suggested in younger infants. This product may increase prolactin levels and, therefore, increase breastmilk production, but it is too hazardous to the infant to use for this purpose. See promethazine as a safer alternative.

Relative infant dose:
Time to clear: Between 1.5 and 4 days
Lactation risk category: L3
Pregnancy risk category: C
Adult dose: 5-10 milligrams three to four times daily
Alternatives: Promethazine

PROGESTERONE

Trade names: Crinone, Prometrium, Gesterol, Cyclogest, Gestone

AAP recommendation: Maternal medication usually compatible with breastfeeding

Progesterone is a naturally occurring steroid (progestin) that is secreted by the ovary, placenta, and adrenal gland. As progesterone is virtually unabsorbed when taken by mouth, the vaginal route has become the most established way to deliver natural progesterone - it is easily administered, avoids liver first-pass metabolism, and has few systemic side-effects. In general, there is of lot of confusion in the literature about the effect of progestins on breastmilk composition.

The changes in breastmilk composition do not appear to be major. With progesterone use, milk volume is normal or higher. Some authors report minor changes in lipid and protein content. However, the majority of the studies were done with other progestins (e.g. medroxyprogesterone). One study found no changes in the development of the infant or breastfeeding performance of study participants who had an intravaginal progesterone ring. The author suggests the ring adds a measure of safety because the amount of steroid present in breastmilk would not be effectively absorbed from the infant's gut.

The effect of progesterones on milk production is poorly studied. Taking progestins in the early postpartum period may actually slow breastmilk production just as it does in pregnant women. It is advisable to wait as long as possible after birth before starting progesterone therapy to avoid reducing the breastmilk supply. The effect of progesterone therapy on the nursing infant is generally unknown, but it is believed minimal to none as natural progesterone is poorly bioavailable to the infant. Several cases of gynecomastia (development of breasts) in infants have been reported but are extremely rare.

Relative infant dose:
Time to clear: Between 2 and 4 days
Lactation risk category: L3
Pregnancy risk category:
Adult dose: 90 milligrams daily
Alternatives:

PROMETHAZINE

Trade names: Phenergan, Promethegan, Avomine, PMS Promethazine

AAP recommendation: Not reviewed

Promethazine is an antihistamine that is primarily used for nausea, vomiting, and motion sickness. It has been used safely for many years in adult and pediatric patients for vomiting, particularly associated with pregnancy. There are no reports on the transfer of promethazine into breastmilk, but small amounts probably do transfer. This product has been used for years for many pediatric conditions. However, recently the FDA has issued warnings about its use in infants due to sedation and apnea. Observe for sedation, particularly in younger infants. Do not use in infants with breathing difficulties (apnea). Long term followup (6 years) has found no harmful effects on development.

Relative infant dose:
Time to clear: Between 2 and 2.5 days
Lactation risk category: L2
Pregnancy risk category: C
Adult dose: 12.5-25 milligrams every 4-6 hours
Alternatives:

PROPOFOL

Trade names: Diprivan

AAP recommendation: Not reviewed

Propofol is an intravenous, sedative, hypnotic anesthetic. It is particularly popular in various pediatric procedures. Although the elimination half-life is long, it is rapidly eliminated from the plasma compartment to other body compartments (fat tissue) so that anesthesia is short (3-10 minutes). Only very low amounts of propofol have been found in breastmilk. There are no reports on the oral absorption of propofol, so we don't know if an infant would absorb it. Propofol is rapidly cleared from the neonatal circulation and is probably safe for use in breastfeeding mothers. A single pumping and discarding of milk at 2-4 hours following surgery would eliminate most risks.

Relative infant dose: 4.4%
Time to clear: Between 4 and 15 days
Lactation risk category: L2
Pregnancy risk category: B

Adult dose: 6-12 milligrams per kilogram per hour
Alternatives: Midazolam

PROPOXYPHENE

Trade names: Darvocet N, Propacet, Darvon, Capadex,
                   Novo-Propoxyn, Dextropropoxyphene, Paradex, Di-Gesic,
                   Doloxene, Progesic
AAP recommendation: Maternal medication usually compatible with
                          breastfeeding

Propoxyphene is a mild narcotic pain killer similar in effectiveness to aspirin. The amount secreted into breastmilk is extremely low, generally too low to produce effects in an infant. Maternal plasma levels peak at 2 hours. So far, harmful effects in infants have not been reported.

Relative infant dose:
Time to clear: Between 1 and 2.5 days
Lactation risk category: L2
Pregnancy risk category: C
Adult dose: 65 milligrams every 4 hours as needed
Alternatives: Ibuprofen, Acetaminophen

PROPRANOLOL

Trade names: Inderal, Novo-Pranol, Deralin, Cardinol
AAP recommendation: Maternal medication usually compatible with
                          breastfeeding

Propranolol is part of the beta-blocker family of drugs and is used to treat high blood pressure, cardiac arrhythmia (abnormal heart rhythm), migraine headaches, and numerous other syndromes. In general, the maternal plasma levels are exceedingly low, thus the breastmilk levels are low as well (less than 0.1% of the maternal dose). The amount of propranolol found in breastmilk would likely be clinically insignificant. One study found no symptoms or signs of beta blockage in the infant. Long-term exposure has not been studied, and some caution is urged. Of the beta blocker family, propranolol (or metoprolol) is probably preferred in lactating women.

Relative infant dose: 0.3%
Time to clear: Between 12 and 25 hours
Lactation risk category: L2

Pregnancy risk category: C
Adult dose: 160-240 milligrams daily
Alternatives: Metoprolol

PROPYLTHIOURACIL

Trade names: PTU

AAP recommendation: Maternal medication usually compatible with breastfeeding

Propylthiouracil is used to treat hyperthyroidism (overactive thyroid gland). Only small amounts of propylthiouracil are secreted into breastmilk. Reports suggest that levels absorbed by the infant are too low to produce suppression of the infant's thyroid. No changes in infant thyroid have been reported in numerous studies. Propylthiouracil is the best antithyroid medication for use in lactating mothers. The infant's thyroid function (T4, TSH) may need to be occassionally monitored during therapy just to be safe, but its not mandatory.

Relative infant dose: 1.8%
Time to clear: Between 4 and 10 hours
Lactation risk category: L2
Pregnancy risk category: D
Adult dose: 100 milligrams three times daily
Alternatives:

PSEUDOEPHEDRINE

Trade names: Sudafed, Halofed, Novafed, Pseudofrin, Balminil, Contac

AAP recommendation: Maternal medication usually compatible with breastfeeding

Pseudoephedrine is primarily used as a nasal decongestant. Pseudoephedrine is secreted into breastmilk in low levels. A recent study found that pseudoephedrine may reduce milk production in some mothers. Mothers in late-stage lactation (more than 12 months postpartum) may be more sensitive to pseudoephedrine and have greater loss of breastmilk production. Therefore, breastfeeding mothers with poor or marginal breastmilk production should be exceedingly cautious in using pseudoephedrine. The amount of pseudoephedrine transferred to the infant via milk is minimal.

Relative infant dose: 4.3%
Time to clear: Between 16 and 20 hours
Lactation risk category: L3 for acute use
L4 for chronic use
Pregnancy risk category: C
Adult dose: 60 milligrams every 4-6 hours
Alternatives:

PYRANTEL

Trade names: Pin-Rid, Reese's Pinworm, Antiminth, Pin-X, Early Bird

AAP recommendation: Not reviewed

Pyrantel is an anthelmintic used to treat pinworm, hookworm and round worm infestations. It is only minimally absorbed orally. The majority is eliminated in feces. It is usually administered as a single dose. Reported side effects are few and minimal. There are no reports on the transfer of pyrantel into breastmilk. Due to minimal oral absorption and low plasma levels, it is unlikely that breastmilk levels would be clinically relevant.

Relative infant dose:
Time to clear:
Lactation risk category: L3
Pregnancy risk category: C
Adult dose: 11 milligrams per kilogram twice over two weeks
Alternatives:

PYRIDOXINE

Trade names: Vitamin B-6, Pyroxin, Complomint continus, Hexa-betalin

AAP recommendation: Maternal medication usually compatible with breastfeeding

Pyridoxine is vitamin B-6. The recommended daily allowance for non-pregnant women is 1.6 milligrams per day. One study clearly indicates that pyridoxine readily transfers into breastmilk and that B-6 levels in milk correlate closely with maternal intake. Greater amounts of pyridoxine are required during pregnancy and lactation. Most prenatal vitamin supplements contain from 12 - 25 milligrams. Very high doses (600 milligrams per day) suppress prolactin secretion and may, therefore, reduce breastmilk production. It is not advisable to take more than 25 milligrams per day.

Relative infant dose:
Time to clear: Between 60 and 100 days
Lactation risk category: L2
                                    L4 in high doses
Pregnancy risk category: A
Adult dose: 1.6 milligrams daily
Alternatives:

QUAZEPAM

Trade names: Doral, Dormalin

AAP recommendation: Drug whose effect on nursing infants is
                                     unknown but may be of concern

Quazepam is part of the "Valium" family of drugs and is used as a sedative.
The authors of one study suggested that very low levels (0.19%) of the
maternal dose would be transferred into breastmilk over a 24 hour period.

Relative infant dose: 0.2%
Time to clear: Between 6.5 and 8 days
Lactation risk category: L2
Pregnancy risk category: X
Adult dose: 15 milligrams daily
Alternatives: Lorazepam, Alprazolam

QUETIAPINE FUMARATE

Trade names: Seroquel

AAP recommendation: Not reviewed

Quetiapine (Seroquel) is indicated for the treatment of psychotic disorders.
It can cause sedation. It has been shown that quetiapine increases prolactin
levels and the incidence of seizures, and lowers thyroid levels in adults. At
present, there are no reports on the transfer of quetiapine into breastmilk.
Until we know more, this product should be considered risky for breastfeeding
women. See risperidone as an alternative.

Relative infant dose:
Time to clear: Between 24 and 30 hours
Lactation risk category: L4
Pregnancy risk category: C

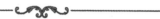
Adult dose: 300-400 milligrams daily
Alternatives:

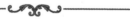

QUINACRINE

Trade names: Atabrine

AAP recommendation: Not reviewed

Quinacrine was once used for malaria, but has been replaced by other drugs. It is now primarily used for giardiasis (protozoa infection). Small to trace amounts of quinacrine are secreted into breastmilk. There are no known harmful effects, except in infants with glucose-6-phosphate dehydrogenase (G6PD) deficiencies. Quinacrine is removed from the body very slowly, requiring up to 2 months for complete removal. Quinacrine levels in the liver are extremely high. A build-up of this drug in the infant is likely due to the slow rate of removal. Caution is urged.

Relative infant dose:
Time to clear: Between 20 and 25 days
Lactation risk category: L4
Pregnancy risk category: C
Adult dose: 100 milligrams three times daily
Alternatives:

QUINAPRIL

Trade names: Accupril, Accuretic, Asig, Accupro

AAP recommendation: Not reviewed

Quinapril is an angiotensin converting enzyme inhibitor (ACE). It is used to lower high blood pressure. The product Accuretic also contains the diuretic hydrochlorothiazide. In one study of women receiving 20 milligrams of quinapril per day, no quinapril or quinaprilat were found in breastmilk. The estimated "dose" of quinapril that would be received by the infant was 1.6% of the maternal dose. The authors suggest that quinapril appears to be safe during breastfeeding; although, a risk:benefit assessment is required. ACE inhibitors are generally not used during pregnancy due to increased harmful effects in the fetus and should not be used by mothers breastfeeding premature infants.

Relative infant dose: 1.6%
Time to clear: Between 8 and 10 hours

Lactation risk category: L2
                                   L4 if used early postpartum
Pregnancy risk category: D
Adult dose: 20-80 milligrams daily
Alternatives: Captopril, Enalapril

QUINIDINE

Trade names: Quinaglute, Quinidex, Cardioquin, Kiditard, Novo-Quinidin, Kinidin Durules

AAP recommendation: Maternal medication usually compatible with breastfeeding

Quinidine is used to treat cardiac arrhythmias (abnormal heart rhythm). Quinidine is selectively stored in the liver, and is transferred into breastmilk at low levels. Long-term use could expose an infant to liver toxicity, but this is unlikely. The infant's liver enzymes should be monitored if it is used chronically in the mother.

Relative infant dose: 14.4%
Time to clear: Between 1 and 1.5 days
Lactation risk category: L2
Pregnancy risk category: C
Adult dose: 200-400 milligrams three to four times daily
Alternatives:

QUININE

Trade names: Quinamm, Biquinate, Myoquin, Quinbisul, Quinate

AAP recommendation: Maternal medication usually compatible with breastfeeding

Quinine is primarily used to prevent and treat malaria. In a study of 6 women, only small to trace amounts of quinine were secreted into breastmilk. The authors suggested these levels were clinically insignificant. No reports of harmful effects have been reported except in infants with glucose-6-phosphate dehydrogenase deficiency (G6PD).

Relative infant dose: 1.3%
Time to clear: Between 44 and 55 hours
Lactation risk category: L2

Pregnancy risk category: D
Adult dose: 650 milligrams every 8 hours
Alternatives:

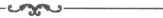

RABEPRAZOLE

Trade names: Aciphex

AAP recommendation: Not reviewed

Rabeprazole is used to treat gastric ulcers among other uses and is similar to omeprazole (Prilosec). There are no reports on levels in breastmilk. Rabeprazole is only 52% bioavailable in adults when enteric coated due to its instability in gastric acids. If rabeprazole is present in breastmilk, it would be virtually destroyed in the infant's stomach prior to absorption.

Relative infant dose:
Time to clear: Between 4 and 10 hours
Lactation risk category: L3
Pregnancy risk category: B
Adult dose: 20 milligrams daily
Alternatives: Omeprazole

RABIES INFECTION

Trade names:

AAP recommendation: Not reviewed

Rabies is an acute, rapidly progressing illness caused by a virus that is usually fatal. Infection is caused by other warm-blooded mammals. Incubation is prolonged and can be up to 4-6 weeks. The virus is seldom found in the blood, but stays in neurologic tissue. Person to person transmission has not been documented nor has there been documentation of transmission of the rabies virus into breastmilk. If a breastfeeding women is exposed to the rabies virus, she should receive the human rabies immune globulin and begin the vaccination series. Most sources agree that once immunization has begun, the mother can continue breastfeeding.

Relative infant dose:
Time to clear:
Lactation risk category:
Pregnancy risk category:
Adult dose:

Alternatives:

RAMIPRIL

Trade names: Altace, Ramace, Tritace
AAP recommendation: Not reviewed

Ramipril is a potent antihypertensive of the ACE inhibitor family. It is used in the management of high blood pressure. ACE inhibitors can cause increased fetal and neonatal morbidity and should never be used in pregnant women. However, ingestion of a single 10 milligram oral dose in a breastfeeding woman produced an undetectable level in breastmilk. Only 0.25% of the total dose is estimated to penetrate into breastmilk. This product should not be used in pregnant woman or women breastfeeding premature infants.

Relative infant dose:	0.3%
Time to clear:	Between 2 and 3.5 days
Lactation risk category:	L3
Pregnancy risk category:	D
Adult dose:	2.5-20 milligrams daily
Alternatives:	Captopril, Enalapril

RANITIDINE

Trade names: Zantac, Novo-Ranidine, Nu-Ranit
AAP recommendation: Not reviewed

Ranitidine reduces acid secretion in the stomach. It has been widely used in pediatrics primarily for gastroesophageal reflux (GER) without significant side effects. The amount transferred into milk is too low to produce clinical effects in the breastfed infant. An infant would ingest at most 0.4 milligrams per kilogram of body weight per day. This amount is quite small considering the pediatric dose currently recommended is 2-4 milligrams per kilogram per day. See nizatidine or famotidine for alternatives.

Relative infant dose:	4.6%
Time to clear:	Between 8 and 15 hours
Lactation risk category:	L2
Pregnancy risk category:	B
Adult dose:	150 milligrams twice daily
Alternatives:	Famotidine, Nizatidine

REPAGLINIDE

Trade names: Prandin, Novonorm

AAP recommendation: Not reviewed

Repaglinide is used to treat non-insulin dependent diabetes mellitus (Type 2). There are no reports on the transfer of repaglinide into breastmilk. Dosing of repaglinide is rather unique, with doses taken prior to each meal due to its short half-life. At this point, we do not know if it is safe for use in breastfeeding patients. If it is used, the infant should be closely monitored for hypoglycemia (low blood sugar) and should not be fed for several hours after the dose to reduce exposure.

Relative infant dose:
Time to clear: Between 4 and 5 hours
Lactation risk category: L4
Pregnancy risk category: C
Adult dose: 0.5-4 milligrams two to four times daily
Alternatives:

RHO (D) IMMUNE GLOBULIN

Trade names: Rhogam, Gamulin RH, Hyprho-D,
                 Mini-Gamulin RH

AAP recommendation: Not reviewed

RHO(D) immune globulin is an immune globulin that contains high concentrations of Rh antibodies. Only trace amounts of anti-Rh were present in colostrum and only low levels in mature breastmilk were found in women receiving large doses of Rh immune globulin. No harmful effects have been reported. Most immunoglobulins are destroyed in the gastric acidity of the newborn infant's stomach. Rh immune globulins are not contraindicated in breastfeeding mothers.

Relative infant dose:
Time to clear: Between 96 and 120 days
Lactation risk category: L2
Pregnancy risk category:
Adult dose: 300 micrograms one to two times
Alternatives:

RIBAVIRIN

Trade names: Virazole, Rebetol, Virazide

AAP recommendation: Not reviewed

Ribavirin is used as an antiviral agent and is effective in a wide variety of viral infections. Its use in breastfeeding patients for treatment of Hepatitis C infections [combined with interferon alfa (Rebetron)] for periods up to one year may be problematic as high concentrations of ribavirin could accumulate in the breastfed infant. There are no reports on its transfer into breastmilk, but it is probably low. Its oral bioavailability is low as well. It is likely that acute (short-term) exposure of a breastfed infant would produce minimal side effects. However, chronic exposure over 6-12 months may be more risky, so caution is recommended.

Relative infant dose:
Time to clear: Between 49.5 and 62 days
Lactation risk category: L4
Pregnancy risk category: X
Adult dose: If less than 165 lb then, 400 milligrams in the
                morning and 600 milligrams in the evening. If more than
                165 lb, then 600 millgrams in the morning and
                evening.

Alternatives:

RIBAVIRIN AND
INTERFERON ALFA-2B

Trade names: Rebetron

AAP recommendation: Not reviewed

Rebetron combines the antiviral drug, Ribavirin, and the immunomodulator drug, interferon alfa-2b. This product is used for the long-term treatment of hepatitis C. Rebetron is extremely dangerous to a fetus and may cause birth defects. Pregnancy must be strictly avoided if this product is used in either the male or female partner. Due to the long half-life of this product, pregnancy should be avoided for at least 6 months following use.

Very little is known about the secretion of interferons in breastmilk; although, some interferons are known to be secreted into breastmilk normally and may contribute to the antiviral properties of breastmilk. Interferons are large in molecular weight which would limit their transfer into breastmilk. One study observed no change in breastmilk levels after a massive dose of interferon alpha was given to a breastfeeding mother. It is unlikely that the interferon in Rebetron would transfer to breastmilk or the infant in clinically relevant amounts. There are no reports on the transfer of Ribavirin + Interferon Alfa 2B into breastmilk, but it is probably low. Its oral bioavailability is low as well. It is likely that acute exposure of a breastfed infant would produce minimal side effects. However, chronic exposure over 12 months may be more risky, so caution is recommended.

Relative infant dose:
Time to clear: Between 49.5 and 62 days
Lactation risk category: L4
Pregnancy risk category: X
Adult dose: If patient weighs less than 165 lb: 3 million IU (international units) interferon alfa 3 times per week with 400 and 600 milligrams ribavirin in the morning and afternoon respectively. If patient weighs more than 165 lb; 3 million IU interferon alpha 3 times per week with 600 milligrams ribavirin twice per day.
Alternatives:

RIMANTADINE HCL

Trade names: Flumadine
AAP recommendation: Not reviewed

Rimantadine is an antiviral agent primarily used for influenza A infections. Rimantadine is transferred into breastmilk in high levels. The manufacturer alludes to toxic side effects, but fails to state them. No side effects have yet been reported in breastfeeding infants. Rimantadine is, however, used to prevent influenza A in pediatric patients less than 1 year of age.

Relative infant dose:
Time to clear: Between 4 and 5.5 days
Lactation risk category: L3
Pregnancy risk category: C
Adult dose: 100 milligrams twice daily
Alternatives:

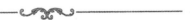

RISEDRONATE

Trade names: Actonel
AAP recommendation: Not reviewed

Risedronate is used in the management of certain syndromes such as Paget's syndrome. Its entry into breastmilk is possible due to its small molecular weight, but it has not yet been reported. Due to the presence of fat and calcium in milk, its oral bioavailability in infants would be exceedingly low. However, the presence of this product in an infant's growing bones is concerning. Some caution is recommended.

Relative infant dose:
Time to clear: Between 80 and 100 days
Lactation risk category: L3
Pregnancy risk category: C
Adult dose: 30 milligrams per day for 2 months
Alternatives:

RISPERIDONE

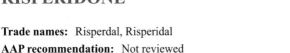

Trade names: Risperdal, Risperidal
AAP recommendation: Not reviewed

Risperidone is a potent antipsychotic agent. Based on studies, risperidone has been detected in breastmilk in small amounts, but was undetectable in the infants' blood. The estimated daily dose of risperidone and metabolite (risperidone equivalents) was 2.8-4.7% of the mother's dose. No harmful effects were noted in the breastfed infants.

Relative infant dose: 2.8%
Time to clear: Between 12 hours and 4 days
Lactation risk category: L3
Pregnancy risk category: C
Adult dose: 3 milligrams twice daily
Alternatives:

RIZATRIPTAN

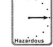

Trade names: Maxalt
AAP recommendation: Not reviewed

Rizatriptan is used in the management of migraine headaches. It is similar in effect to sumatriptan. There are no reports on the transfer of rizatriptan into breastmilk. The kinetics of this drug may predispose it to higher breastmilk levels. Sumatriptan is preferred at this time.

Relative infant dose:
Time to clear: Between 8 and 15 hours

Lactation risk category: L3
Pregnancy risk category: C
Adult dose: 5-10 milligrams by mouth, repeat only after 2 hours
Alternatives: Sumatriptan

ROPIVACAINE

Trade names: Naropin

AAP recommendation: Not reviewed

Ropivacaine is a newer local anesthetic commonly used as a regional anesthetic and for epidural drips. It is believed to produce fewer complications, such as low blood pressure, when compared to bupivacaine. There are no reports on the transfer of ropivacaine into breastmilk, but the manufacturer suggests it is probably much lower than the infant receives in utero. This agent is commonly used in obstetrics and probably poses few, if any problems, to a breastfeeding infant.

Relative infant dose:
Time to clear: Between 17 and 21 hours
Lactation risk category: L2
Pregnancy risk category: B
Adult dose: Epidural = 75-150 milligrams
Alternatives: Bupivacaine

ROSIGLITAZONE

Trade names: Avandia

AAP recommendation: Not reviewed

Rosiglitazone is used in the management of diabetes mellitus. There are no reports on its transfer into breastmilk.

Relative infant dose:
Time to clear: Between 12 and 20 hours
Lactation risk category: L3
Pregnancy risk category: C
Adult dose: 2-8 milligrams daily
Alternatives:

SACCHARIN

Trade names:

AAP recommendation: Not reviewed

Saccharin is an artificial sweetener. One study of 6 women suggested milk levels were low. After repeated dosing, saccharin appears to accumulate over time. Moderate intake of saccarin should be compatible with breastfeeding.

Relative infant dose:	3.7%
Time to clear:	Between 19.5 and 24 hours
Lactation risk category:	L3
Pregnancy risk category:	C
Adult dose:	
Alternatives:	

SAGE

Trade names: Sage, Dalmatian, Spanish

AAP recommendation: Not reviewed

Salvia officinalis L. (Dalmatian sage) and Salvia lavandulaefolia Vahl (Spanish sage) are the most common of the species. Extracts and teas have been used to treat digestive disorders (antispasmodic), as an antiseptic and astringent, and in treating diarrhea, gastritis, sore throat, and other diseases. The dried and smoked leaves have been used to treat asthma symptoms. Sage has also been used to dry up a mother's milk supply. These uses are largely unproven in the literature. Sage extracts have been found to be strong antioxidants with some antimicrobial properties.

For the most part, sage is relatively nontoxic and nonirritating. Ingestion of large quantities may lead to cracking and inflammation of the lips, inflammation of the mouth, dry mouth, or local irritation. Due to the drying properties and pediatric hypersensitivity, sage should be used with some caution in breastfeeding mothers as it can potentially reduce the mother's milk supply.

Relative infant dose:	
Time to clear:	
Lactation risk category:	L4
Pregnancy risk category:	
Adult dose:	
Alternatives:	

SALMETEROL XINAFOATE

Trade names: Serevent

AAP recommendation: Not reviewed

Salmeterol is used to treat asthma. If salmeterol is inhaled, maternal plasma levels of salmeterol are undetectable making the risk to the infant very low. Oral absorption of both the salmeterol and the xinafoate moiety are good. There are no reports of use in breastfeeding women.

Relative infant dose:
Time to clear: Between 22 and 27.5 hours
Lactation risk category: L2
Pregnancy risk category: C
Adult dose: 50 micrograms twice daily
Alternatives:

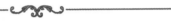

SCOPOLAMINE

Trade names: Transderm Scope, Buscopan, Benacine,
                    Scopoderm TTS

AAP recommendation: Maternal medication usually compatible with
                    breastfeeding

Scopolamine is used mainly for motion sickness and to produce amnesia and decrease salivation before an operation. Scopolamine is structurally similar to atropine, but is known for its prominent central nervous system effects. There are no reports on its transfer into breastmilk. Due to its poor oral absorption, transfer is generally believed to be minimal.

Relative infant dose:
Time to clear: Between 11.5 and 14.5 hours
Lactation risk category: L3
Pregnancy risk category: C
Adult dose: 0.3-0.6 milligrams once
Alternatives:

SECOBARBITAL

Trade names: Seconal, Seconal sodium

AAP recommendation: Maternal medication usually compatible with breastfeeding

Secobarbital is part of the barbiturate family of drugs It is a sedative and hypnotic. It is probably secreted into breastmilk; although, levels are unknown. It can be found in breastmilk for 24 hours or longer. It is recommended that mothers delay breastfeeding for 3-4 hours after taking secobarbital to reduce possible transfer to infant if exposure to secobarbital is required.

Relative infant dose:
Time to clear: Between 2.5 and 8.5 days
Lactation risk category: L3
Pregnancy risk category: D
Adult dose: 100 milligrams daily
Alternatives:

SELENIUM SULFIDE

Trade names: Selsun, Head and Shoulders, Selsun Blue, Exsel

AAP recommendation: Not reviewed

Selenium sulfide is an anti-infective compound with mild antibacterial and antifungal activity. It is commonly used for fungal skin infections and dandruff. Selenium is not absorbed in significant amounts through intact skin, but is absorbed through damaged skin or open lesions. There are no reports on the transfer of selenium into breastmilk. If used on undamaged skin, it is unlikely that enough would be absorbed to produce harmful effects in a breastfed infant. Do not apply directly to nipples as this might enhance absorption by the infant.

Relative infant dose:
Time to clear:
Lactation risk category: L3
Pregnancy risk category:
Adult dose: Apply topically twice weekly
Alternatives: Topical Clotrimazole, Ketaconazole shampoo

SENNA LAXATIVES

Trade names: Senokot, Senexon, Ex Lax, Senna-Gen,
Black-Draught, Fletcher's Castoria, Agoral

AAP recommendation: Maternal medication usually compatible with
breastfeeding

Senna is a potent laxative. Anthraquinones, its key ingredients, are believed to increase bowel activity. Side effects such as abdominal cramping and colic are unpredictable with homemade varieties of this plant. Most sources recommend taking a standardized formulation commonly available. This product is only recommended for short term use, such as 10 days. Do not use for intestinal obstruction, appendicitis, or abdominal pain of unknown origin. Senna laxatives are occasionally used in postpartum women to alleviate constipation. In one study of women receiving Senokot (100 milligrams containing 8.602 milligrams of Sennosides A and B), no sennoside A or B was found in their breastmilk and only 2 out of 15 breastfed infants had loose stools.

Relative infant dose:
Time to clear:
Lactation risk category: L3
Pregnancy risk category:
Adult dose: 100 milligrams daily
Alternatives:

SERTRALINE

Trade names: Zoloft, Lustral

AAP recommendation: Drug whose effect on nursing infants is
unknown but may be of concern

Sertraline is an antidepressant similar to Prozac and Paxil. Studies of large numbers of infants/mothers clearly confirm that the transfer of sertraline and its metabolite, desmethylsertraline, to the infant is minimal. Clinically relevant plasma levels in infants is remote at maternal doses less than 150 milligram per day. No harmful effects have been reported and no developmental abnormalities were noted in the breastfed infants. This is the preferred antidepressant for breastfeeding mothers.

Relative infant dose: 2.2%
Time to clear: Between 4.5 and 13.5 days
Lactation risk category: L2
Pregnancy risk category: B

Adult dose: 50-200 milligrams daily
Alternatives: Paroxetine

SILICONE BREAST IMPLANTS

Trade names:
AAP recommendation: Not reviewed

Silicone is found in all foods, liquids, etc. Breast enlargement with silicone implants is now available in the USA. Saline implants are now the standard. In general, placement of the implant behind the breast tissue seldom produces interruption of vital ducts, nerve supply, or blood supply. Most women with breast enlargements have been able to breastfeed. Breast reduction surgery, on the other hand, removes ducts and nerves, and may lead to a reduced ability to lactate. It is not known for certain if ingestion of leaking silicone by a breastfeeding infant is dangerous.

One article showing esophageal strictures was recalled by the author. Silicone by nature is extremely inert and unlikely to be absorbed in the gastrointestinal tract by a nursing infant; although, good studies are lacking. Silicon levels are 10 times higher in cow's milk and even higher in infant formula.

Relative infant dose:
Time to clear:
Lactation risk category:
Pregnancy risk category:
Adult dose:
Alternatives:

SILVER SULFADIAZINE

Trade names: Silvadene, SSD Cream, Thermazene, Dermazin, SSD, Silvazine, Flamazine

AAP recommendation: Not reviewed

Silver sulfadiazine is a topical antimicrobial cream primarily used for reducing sepsis in burn patients. The silver component is not absorbed from the skin. The sulfadiazine is partially absorbed. After prolonged therapy of large areas, sulfadiazine levels in plasma may approach therapeutic levels. Although sulfonamides are known to be secreted into breastmilk, they are not a problem except in the newborn period when they may produce kernicterus (abnormal accumulation of bile pigment in the brain).

Relative infant dose:

Time to clear:	Between 1.5 and 2 days
Lactation risk category:	L3
Pregnancy risk category:	B
Adult dose:	
Alternatives:	

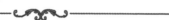

SOTALOL

Trade names: Betapace, Apo-Sotalol, Rylosol, Cardol, Sotacor

AAP recommendation: Maternal medication usually compatible with breastfeeding

Sotalol is a typical beta blocker used to lower high blood pressure. Sotalol is transferred into breastmilk in high levels. Although the reported levels appear high, no evidence of toxicity has been reported.

Relative infant dose:	25.5%
Time to clear:	Between 2 and 2.5 days
Lactation risk category:	L3
Pregnancy risk category:	B
Adult dose:	80-160 milligrams twice daily
Alternatives:	Propranolol, Metoprolol

ST. JOHN'S WORT

Trade names:

AAP recommendation: Not reviewed

St. John's Wort (Hypericum perforatum) consists of the whole fresh or dried plant or its components containing not less than 0.04% naphthodianthrones of the hypericin group. Hypericum has become increasingly popular for the treatment of depression following results from numerous studies showing effectiveness. Patients taking anticonvulsants and other critically important drugs should be advised about the possible interaction with St. John's wort leading to major reductions in plasma levels of other drugs.

Patients should always advise their physicians of their use of St. John's Wort. In one study, hyperforin but not hypericin was detected at very low levels in breastmilk of lactating mothers. Both components were undetectable in the blood of the infant. No side effects of any kind were noted in the infant and the Denver Developmental Screen was normal.

Relative infant dose:
Time to clear: Between 4.5 and 5.5 days
Lactation risk category: L2
Pregnancy risk category:
Adult dose: 300 milligrams three times daily dry-powdered (0.3% hypericin)
Alternatives: Sertraline, Paroxetine

SUCRALFATE

Trade names: Carafate, Novo-Sucralfate, Nu-Sucralfate, Carafate, SCF, Ulcyte, Antepsin

AAP recommendation: Not reviewed

Sucralfate is a sucrose aluminum complex used for stomach ulcers. When taken orally, sucralfate forms a complex that physically covers stomach ulcers. Less than 5% is absorbed orally. At these plasma levels, it is very unlikely to penetrate into breastmilk.

Relative infant dose:
Time to clear:
Lactation risk category: L2
Pregnancy risk category: B
Adult dose: 1 gram four times daily
Alternatives:

SULCONAZOLE NITRATE

Trade names: Exelderm

AAP recommendation: Not reviewed

Sulconazole (Exelderm) is an antifungal topical cream. Although there are no reports on the transfer of sulconazole into breastmilk, it is unlikely that the degree of transdermal absorption would be high enough to produce significant milk levels. Only 8.7% of the topically administered dose is absorbed through the skin.

Relative infant dose:
Time to clear:
Lactation risk category: L3
Pregnancy risk category: C
Adult dose: Topical

Alternatives:

SULFAMETHOXAZOLE

Trade names: Gantanol, Bactrim, Resprim, Septrin
AAP recommendation: Not reviewed

Sulfamethoxazole is a common and popular antibiotic that is transferred into breastmilk in small amounts. Use with caution in weakened infants, premature infants, or neonates with high bilirubin levels. Gantrisin (Sulfisoxazole) is considered the best choice of sulfonamides due to reduced transfer to the infant. This drug is compatible with breastfeeding but exercise caution.

Relative infant dose:
Time to clear: Between 1.5 and 2 days
Lactation risk category: L3
Pregnancy risk category: C
Adult dose: 1-2 grams twice daily
Alternatives:

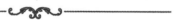

SULFASALAZINE

Trade names: Azulfidine, Salazopyrin, SAS-500
AAP recommendation: Drug associated with significant side effects and should be taken with caution

Sulfasalazine is used as an anti-inflammatory for ulcerative colitis. Only one-third of the dose is absorbed by the mother and most of the dose stays in the gastrointestinal tract. Secretion of 5-aminosalicylic acid (active compound) and its inactive metabolite (acetyl -5-ASA) into breastmilk is very low. Few if any adverse effects have been observed in most nursing infants. However, there has been one reported case of toxicity which may have been an allergic response peculiar to the individual. Use with caution.

Relative infant dose: 0.4%
Time to clear: Between 1 and 1.5 days
Lactation risk category: L3
Pregnancy risk category: B
Adult dose: 500 milligrams every 6 hours
Alternatives:

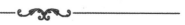

SULFISOXAZOLE

Trade names: Gantrisin, Azo-Gantrisin, Sulfizole

AAP recommendation: Maternal medication usually compatible with breastfeeding

Sulfisoxazole is a popular antibiotic and is part of the sulfonamide family of drugs. Sulfisoxazole is transferred into breastmilk in small amounts; although, the actual levels are somewhat controversial. Less than 1% of the maternal dose is transferred into breastmilk. This is probably insufficient to produce problems in a normal newborn. Sulfisoxazole appears to be the best choice. Use with caution in weakened infants or those with high blood levels of bilirubin.

Relative infant dose:
Time to clear: Between 18.5 and 39 hours
Lactation risk category: L2
Pregnancy risk category: C
Adult dose: 1-4 grams every 4-6 hours
Alternatives:

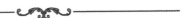

SUMATRIPTAN SUCCINATE

Trade names: Imitrex, Imigran

AAP recommendation: Maternal medication usually compatible with breastfeeding

Sumatriptan is used to treat migraine headaches. Sumatriptan is not a pain killer. In one study, the maternal plasma levels of sumatriptan was small with low milk concentrations. The total recovery of sumatriptan in milk over 8 hours was only 3.5% of the maternal dose. The authors suggest that continued breastfeeding following sumatriptan use would not pose a significant risk to the infant.

Relative infant dose: 3.5%
Time to clear: Between 5 and 6.5 hours
Lactation risk category: L3
Pregnancy risk category: C
Adult dose: 25-100 milligrams two to three times daily

Alternatives:

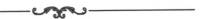

TAZAROTENE

Trade names: Tazorac, Zorac

AAP recommendation: Not reviewed

Tazarotene is used for the topical treatment of stable plaque psoriasis (reddish, silvery-scaled lesions which occur mainly on the elbows, knees, scalp and trunk) and acne. Following topical application, tazarotene is converted to its active metabolite, tazarotenic acid. Absorption from the skin is minimal (less than 1%). Little of the compound could be detected in the plasma. When applied to large surface areas, systemic absorption is increased. There are no reports on the transfer into breastmilk, but it is unlikely.

Relative infant dose:
Time to clear: Between 72 and 90 hours
Lactation risk category: L3
Pregnancy risk category: X
Adult dose: Apply daily
Alternatives:

TEA TREE OIL

Trade names:

AAP recommendation: Not reviewed

Tea tree oil, as derived from Melaleuca alternifolia, has recently gained popularity for its antiseptic properties. Tea tree oil is primarily noted for its antimicrobial effects without irritating sensitive tissues. In several reports, it is suggested to have antifungal properties equivalent to tolnaftate and clotrimazole. Although the use of tea tree oil in adults is mostly nontoxic, the safe use in infants is unknown. Use directly on the nipple should be minimized.

Relative infant dose:
Time to clear:
Lactation risk category: L3
Pregnancy risk category:
Adult dose:
Alternatives:

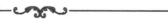

TEGASEROD MALEATE

Trade names: Zelnorm

AAP recommendation: Not reviewed

Tegaserod is used to treat the symptoms of irritable bowel syndrome. Oral absorption is only 10% (fasting) and is reduced 40-65% if taken with food. There are no reports on the transfer of tegaserod into breastmilk. Tegaserod is a lipophilic drug which would assist its transfer into breastmilk, however, its low plasma levels, poor oral absorption (particularly with food), and large volume of distribution suggests that the actual amount transferred into breastmilk and absorbed by the infant is probably quite low.

Relative infant dose:
Time to clear: Between 44 and 55 hours
Lactation risk category: L3
Pregnancy risk category: B
Adult dose: 6 milligrams twice daily
Alternatives:

TELMISARTAN

Trade names: Micardis, Micardis HCT

AAP recommendation: Not reviewed

Telmisartan is used to lower high blood pressure. Micardis HCT also contains 12.5 milligrams hydrochlorothiazide (diuretic). This drug should never be used in pregnant patients as fetal death has been reported with similar agents in this class. There are no reports on the use of telmisartan in lactating mothers. It should not be used in mothers with premature infants.

Relative infant dose:
Time to clear: Between 4 and 5 days
Lactation risk category: L3
                                L4 if used in neonatal period
Pregnancy risk category: C during 1st and 2nd trimesters
                                D during 3rd trimester
Adult dose: 40 milligrams daily
Alternatives:

TEMAZEPAM

Trade names: Restoril, PMS-Temazepam, Euhypnos, Noctume, Temaze, Temtabs, Normison

AAP recommendation: Drug whose effect on nursing infants is unknown but may be of concern

Temazepam is a part of the "Valium" family of drugs. It is used as a nighttime sedative. Temazepam is relatively water soluble and, therefore, transfers poorly into breastmilk. Levels of temazepam were undetectable in the infants studied; although, these studies were carried out 15 hours post-dose. Although the study shows low neonatal exposure to temazepam via breastmilk, the infant should be monitored carefully for sleepiness and poor feeding.

Relative infant dose:
Time to clear: Between 1.5 and 2.5 days
Lactation risk category: L3
Pregnancy risk category: X
Adult dose: 7.5-30 milligrams daily
Alternatives: Lorazepam, Alprazolam

TERBINAFINE

Trade names: Lamisil

AAP recommendation: Not reviewed

Terbinafine is an antifungal agent primarily used to treat athlete's foot and ringworm. Systemic absorption following topical therapy is minimal. Topical absorption through the skin is minimal. The total excretion of terbinafine in breastmilk ranges from 0.13% to 0.03% of the total maternal dose respectively.

Relative infant dose:
Time to clear: Between 4.5 and 5.5 days
Lactation risk category: L2
Pregnancy risk category: B
Adult dose: 250 milligrams daily
Alternatives: Fluconazole

TERBUTALINE

Trade names: Bricanyl, Brethine

AAP recommendation: Maternal medication usually compatible with breastfeeding

Terbutaline is used for the symptomatic relief of asthma and is transferred into breastmilk in low quantities. Only 0.2 to 0.7% of the maternal dose is likely to be transferred to the infant via breastmilk. In one study, terbutaline was not detectable in the infant's serum. No harmful effects have been reported in breastfeeding infants.

Relative infant dose: 0.2%
Time to clear: Between 2.5 and 3 days
Lactation risk category: L2
Pregnancy risk category: B
Adult dose: 5 milligrams three times daily
Alternatives:

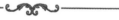

TERCONAZOLE

Trade names: Terazol 3, Terazol 7

AAP recommendation: Not reviewed

Terconazole is an antifungal primarily used for vaginal candidiasis. It is similar to fluconazole and itraconazole. When terconazole is administered intravaginally, only a limited amount (5 -16%) is absorbed systemically. Terconazole is well absorbed orally. Even at high doses, the drug is not mutagenic or hazardous to the fetus. There are no reports on the transfer of terconazole into breastmilk. The breastmilk levels are probably too small to be clinically relevant.

Relative infant dose:
Time to clear: Between 16 hours and 2.5 days
Lactation risk category: L3
Pregnancy risk category: C
Adult dose: 5 grams daily
Alternatives: Fluconazole

TETRACYCLINE

Trade names: Achromycin, Sumycin, Terramycin,
Tetracyn, Aureomycin, Mysteclin, Tetrex, Tetrachel

AAP recommendation: Maternal medication usually compatible with breastfeeding

Tetracycline is an antibiotic with significant side effects in pediatric patients, including dental staining and reduced bone growth. It is transferred into breastmilk in extremely small amounts. Because tetracyclines bind to breastmilk calcium, they would have reduced oral absorption in the infant. In at least three studies, the relative infant dose varies from 0.6%, 4.77% and 8.44%. Thus a high degree of variability exists in these studies. Mixing tetracyclines in milk would greatly limit their oral bioavailability. The short-term exposure (less than 3 weeks) of infants to tetracyclines (via breastmilk) is not contraindicated.

The authors do not recommend the long-term exposure of breastfeeding infants to tetracyclines such as when used daily for acne. The absorption of even small amounts over a prolonged period could result in dental staining.

Relative infant dose: 0.6%
Time to clear: Between 1 and 2.5 days
Lactation risk category: L2
Pregnancy risk category: D
Adult dose: 500 milligrams four times daily
Alternatives:

THEOPHYLLINE

Trade names: Aminophylline, Quibron, Theo-Dur, Austyn,
Pulmophylline, Quibron-T/SR, Nuelin

AAP recommendation: Maternal medication usually compatible with breastfeeding

Theophylline is a bronchodilator used in the management of asthma. Theophylline is transferred into breastmilk. It is estimated that less than 1% of the dose is actually absorbed by the infant. The dose transferred into milk would be approximately 5.8% of the maternal dose. One reported case of irritability and fretful sleeping was reported in an infant exposed to breastmilk only on days when the mother reported taking theophylline.

Relative infant dose: 5.8%
Time to clear: Between 12 hours and 2.5 days

Lactation risk category: L3
Pregnancy risk category: C
Adult dose: 3 milligrams per kilogram every 8 hours
Alternatives:

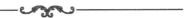

THIABENDAZOLE

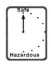

Trade names: Mintezol

AAP recommendation: Not reviewed

Thiabendazole is an antiparasitic agent used to treat roundworm, pinworm, hookworm, whipworm and other parasitic infections. Thiabendazole can be used in children. Although it is effective in treating pinworms, other drugs with fewer side effects are preferred. There are no reports on the transfer of thiabendazole into breastmilk.

Relative infant dose:
Time to clear:
Lactation risk category: L3
Pregnancy risk category: C
Adult dose: 1.5 grams twice daily
Alternatives: Pyrantel

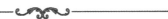

TICARCILLIN

Trade names: Ticar, Timentin, Tarcil, Ticillin

AAP recommendation: Maternal medication usually compatible with breastfeeding

Ticarcillin is part of the penicillin family of antibiotics. Timentin is ticarcillin with clavulanate added. Little is absorbed when taken orally. As with many penicillins, only minimal levels are transferred into breastmilk. Poor oral absorption of ticarcillin would limit exposure of the breastfeeding infant. It may cause changes in gastrointestinal flora and, possibly, fungal overgrowth.

Relative infant dose: 0.2%
Time to clear: Between 3.5 and 6.5 hours
Lactation risk category: L1
Pregnancy risk category: B
Adult dose: 150-300 milligrams daily

Alternatives:

TIMOLOL

Trade names: Blocadren, Timoptic, Novo-Timol, Tenopt,
  Timpilo, Betim, Timoptol

AAP recommendation: Maternal medication usually compatible with
  breastfeeding

Timolol is used to treat high blood pressure and glaucoma. It is transferred into breastmilk, but in amounts too small to be clinically relevant. No harmful effects in infants have been reported.

Relative infant dose: 1.1%
Time to clear: Between 16 and 20 hours
Lactation risk category: L2
Pregnancy risk category: C
Adult dose: 10-20 milligrams twice daily
Alternatives:

TINZAPARIN SODIUM

Trade names: Innohep, Logiparin

AAP recommendation: Not reviewed

Tinzaparin is a heparin derivative used as an anticoagulant. There are no reports on its transfer into breastmilk, but it is probably low. It is very unlikely that any of the above mentioned drug would be orally bioavailable, thus reducing the risk to the infant.

Relative infant dose:
Time to clear: Between 12 and 20 hours
Lactation risk category: L3
Pregnancy risk category: B
Adult dose: 175 IU (international units) per kilogram per day (highly
  variable)
Alternatives: Dalteparin, Enoxaparin

TIZANIDINE

Trade names: Zanaflex

AAP recommendation: Not reviewed

Tizanidine is a muscle relaxant used in the treatment of tension headache and spasticity associated with multiple sclerosis. It is not known if tizanidine transfers into breastmilk. The manufacturer states that due to its lipid solubility, it is likely to penetrate into breastmilk. It has a high rate of sedation (48%) which could be a problem in breastfed infants were they to absorb this medication. Breastfeeding mothers should use this drug with caution.

Relative infant dose:
Time to clear: Between 2 and 4.5 days
Lactation risk category: L4
Pregnancy risk category: C
Adult dose: 8 milligrams every 6 hours as needed
Alternatives:

TOBRAMYCIN

Trade names: Nebcin, Tobrex, Tobi, Tobralex

AAP recommendation: Not reviewed

Tobramycin is an antibiotic similar to gentamicin. Although small levels of tobramycin are known to transfer into breastmilk, they probably pose few problems. Tobramycin is poorly absorbed orally and would be unlikely to produce significant levels in an infant. Observe for diarrhea and change in stool patterns.

Relative infant dose: 6.6%
Time to clear: Between 8 and 15 hours
Lactation risk category: L3
Pregnancy risk category: C
Adult dose: 1 milligram per kilogram every 8 hours
Alternatives:

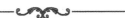

A Medication Guide for Breastfeeding Moms

TOLBUTAMIDE

Trade names: Oramide, Orinase, Mobenol,
Novo-Butamide, Rastinon, Glyconon

AAP recommendation: Maternal medication usually compatible with
breastfeeding

Tolbutamide is used in the management of non-insulin dependent diabetes mellitus (Type 2). Only minimal amounts of tolbutamide are transferred into breastmilk. Observe infant closely for jaundice and low blood sugar.

Relative infant dose: 0.02%
Time to clear: Between 18 and 32.5 hours
Lactation risk category: L3
Pregnancy risk category: D
Adult dose: 250-2000 milligrams daily
Alternatives:

TOLMETIN SODIUM

Trade names: Tolectin

AAP recommendation: Maternal medication usually compatible with
breastfeeding

Tolmetin is a non-steroidal pain killer (NSAID). It is known to be distributed into breastmilk in small amounts. Tolmetin is sometimes used in pediatric rheumatoid arthritis patients (less than 2 years of age). The estimate of dose per day an infant would receive from breastmilk is 115 micrograms per liter of milk.

Relative infant dose: 0.5%
Time to clear: Between 4 and 7.5 hours
Lactation risk category: L3
Pregnancy risk category: C
Adult dose: 200-600 milligrams three times daily
Alternatives: Ibuprofen

TOLTERODINE

Trade names: Detrol, Detrusitol

AAP recommendation: Not reviewed

Tolterodine is used to treat patients with an overactive bladder who have symptoms of urgency, incontinence, or urinary frequency. While we have no reports on the transfer of tolterodine into breastmilk, it is unlikely amounts will be high enough to produce harmful effects in infants. However, the infant should be monitored for symptoms of dehydration - dry mouth, constipation, poor tearing, etc.

Relative infant dose:
Time to clear: Between 7.5 and 18.5 hours
Lactation risk category: L3
Pregnancy risk category: C
Adult dose: 2 milligrams twice daily
Alternatives:

TOPIRAMATE

Trade names: Topamax

AAP recommendation: Not reviewed

Topiramate is a new anticonvulsant used to control seizures. Topiramate has become increasingly popular because it has fewer adverse side effects. The plasma levels found in breastfeeding infants were significantly less than in maternal plasma, making the risk of using this product in breastfeeding mothers probably acceptable. Plasma levels in infants varied from undetectable to low. Close observation of the infant for sedation is advised.

Relative infant dose: 24.5%
Time to clear: Between 3 and 5 days
Lactation risk category: L3
Pregnancy risk category: C
Adult dose: 200 milligrams twice daily
Alternatives:

TRAMADOL HCL

Trade names: Ultram, Ultracet, Tramal, Nycodol, Tramake, Zydol, Zamadol, Dromadol

AAP recommendation: Not reviewed

Tramadol is a new class of pain killer that appears to be slightly more potent than codeine. Ultracet is the combination of tramadol (Ultram) and acetaminophen. See acetominophen. Tramadol enters breastmilk at low levels (0.1% of the maternal dose).

Relative infant dose:
Time to clear: Between 1 and 1.5 days
Lactation risk category: L3
Pregnancy risk category: C
Adult dose: 50-100 milligrams every 4-6 hours as needed
Alternatives: Codeine

TRAZODONE

Trade names: Desyrel, Apo-Trazodone, Molipaxin, Novo-Trazodone, Trazorel

AAP recommendation: Drug whose effect on nursing infants is unknown but may be of concern

Trazodone is an antidepressant. The authors of one study estimated that about 0.6 % of the maternal dose was ingested by the infant over 24 hours. No harmful effects were reported.

Relative infant dose: 0.7%
Time to clear: Between 16 and 45 hours
Lactation risk category: L2
Pregnancy risk category: C
Adult dose: 150-400 milligrams daily
Alternatives:

TRETINOIN

Trade names: Retin-A, Renova, Stieva-A, Vitamin A Acid, Vesanoid

AAP recommendation: Not reviewed

Tretinoin is a retinoid derivative similar to Vitamin A. It is mainly used topically for acne and wrinkling. It is sometimes taken orally for leukemias (cancer of the blood) and psoriasis (reddish, silvery-scaled lesions which occur mainly on the elbows, knees, scalp and trunk). Absorption of topically applied tretinoin (Retin-A) is reported to be minimal and transfer into breastmilk would likely be minimal to none. If it is used orally, transfer into breastmilk is likely and should be used with great caution in a breastfeeding mother.

Relative infant dose:
Time to clear: Between 8 and 10 hours
Lactation risk category: L3
Pregnancy risk category: B for topical Retin A
C for topical Renova
D for oral

Adult dose: Variable
Alternatives:

TRIAMCINOLONE ACETONIDE

Trade names: Nasacort, Azmacort, Tri-Nasal, Kenalog, Triaderm, Aristocort, Kenalone, Adcortyl

AAP recommendation: Not reviewed

Triamcinolone is a typical corticosteroid (see prednisone) that is available for topical, intranasal, injection, inhalation and oral use. When applied topically to the nose (Nasacort) or to the lungs (Azmacort), only minimal doses are used and plasma levels in the mother are exceedingly low to undetectable. Although there are no reports on triamcinolone secretion into breastmilk, it is likely that the milk levels would be exceedingly low and not clinically relevant when administered via inhalation or intranasally. See prednisone for more breastfeeding data.

Relative infant dose:
Time to clear: Between 6 and 7.5 hours
Lactation risk category: L3
Pregnancy risk category: C
Adult dose: 200 micrograms three to four times daily

Alternatives:

TRIAMTERENE

Trade names: Dyazide, Hydrene
AAP recommendation: Not reviewed

Triamterene is a diuretic that increases the flow of urine and is commonly used in combination with other diuretics such as hydrochlorothiazide (Dyazide). There are no reports on the transfer of triamterene into breastmilk. Because of the availability of other less dangerous diuretics, triamterene should be used as a last resort in breastfeeding mothers.

Relative infant dose:
Time to clear: Between 6 and 12.5 hours
Lactation risk category: L3
Pregnancy risk category: B
Adult dose: 25-100 milligrams daily
Alternatives: Hydrochlorothiazide

TRIAZOLAM

Trade names: Halcion, Novo-Triolam
AAP recommendation: Not reviewed

Triazolam is part of the "Valium" family of drugs and is used as a nighttime sedative. There are no reports on the transfer of triazolam into breastmilk. As with all such drugs, some entry into breastmilk is likely.

Relative infant dose:
Time to clear: Between 6 and 27.5 hours
Lactation risk category: L3
Pregnancy risk category: X
Adult dose: 0.125-0.25 milligrams daily
Alternatives: Lorazepam, Alprazolam

TRIMEPRAZINE

Trade names: Temaril, Vallergan

AAP recommendation: Not reviewed

Trimeprazine is an antihistamine from the phenothiazine family. It is used for itching and is secreted into breastmilk in very low levels, although exact amounts have not been reported.

Relative infant dose:
Time to clear: Between 20 and 25 hours
Lactation risk category: L3
Pregnancy risk category: C
Adult dose: 5 milligrams twice daily
Alternatives:

TRIMETHOPRIM

Trade names: Proloprim, Trimpex, Alprim, Triprim, Ipral, Monotrim, Tiempe

AAP recommendation: Maternal medication usually compatible with breastfeeding

Trimethoprim is an antibiotic. It is transferred into breastmilk at low levels. Because it may interfere with folate metabolism, some caution is recommended in premature infants. However, trimethoprim apparently poses few problems in full term or older infants.

Relative infant dose: 9.0%
Time to clear: Between 1 and 2 days
Lactation risk category: L3
Pregnancy risk category: C
Adult dose: 200 milligrams daily
Alternatives:

TRIPELENNAMINE

Trade names: PBZ, Colrex, Tromide

AAP recommendation: Not reviewed

Tripelennamine is an antihistamine. It is generally not recommended in pediatric patients, particularly neonates due to increased sleep apnea (cessation of respiration during sleep). There are no reports on the transfer of tripelennamine into breastmilk. See loratadine as an alternative.

Relative infant dose:
Time to clear: Between 8 and 15 hours
Lactation risk category: L4
Pregnancy risk category: B
Adult dose: 25-50 milligrams every 4-6 hours
Alternatives: Loratadine

TRIPROLIDINE

Trade names: Actidil, Actacin, Actifed, Codral, Pro-Actidil

AAP recommendation: Maternal medication usually compatible with breastfeeding

Triprolidine is an antihistamine. It is marketed with pseudoephedrine as Actifed. The infant dose is less than 1.8% of the maternal dose. This dose is far too low to be clinically relevant.

Relative infant dose: 1.8%
Time to clear: Between 20 and 25 hours
Lactation risk category: L1
Pregnancy risk category: C
Adult dose: 2.5 milligrams every 4-6 hours
Alternatives: Loratadine

TUBERCULIN PURIFIED PROTEIN DERIVATIVE

Trade names: Tubersol, Aplisol, Sclavo, PPD, Mantoux

AAP recommendation: Not reviewed

Tuberculin (also called Mantoux, PPD, Tine test) is a skin-test antigen. Small amounts of this purified product are injected into the skin. It produces a reaction at the injection site in those individuals with antibodies to tuberculosis. Preliminary studies indicate that breast-fed infants may passively acquire sensitivity to mycobacterial antigens from mothers who are sensitized. There are no contraindications to using PPD tests in breastfeeding mothers as the proteins are sterilized and unlikely to penetrate breastmilk.

Relative infant dose:

Time to clear:
Lactation risk category: L2
Pregnancy risk category: C
Adult dose: 5 units once
Alternatives:

URSODIOL

Trade names: Actigall, Combidol, Destolit, Lithofalk, Urdox, Ursogal

AAP recommendation: Not reviewed

Ursodiol (ursodeoxycholic acid) is a bile salt. It is used commercially to dissolve gallbladder stones. It is almost completely absorbed orally. Only trace amounts are found in the plasma. It is not likely that significant amounts would be present in breastmilk. While there are no reports on breastfeeding, only small amounts of bile salts are known to be present in milk.

Relative infant dose:
Time to clear:
Lactation risk category: L3
Pregnancy risk category: B
Adult dose: 8-10 milligrams per kilogram per day in 3 divided doses
Alternatives:

VALACYCLOVIR

Trade names: Valtrex, Valaciclovir

AAP recommendation: Not reviewed

Valacyclovir is a medication that is rapidly metabolized in the plasma to acyclovir. Thus acyclovir is the active ingredient. The amount of acyclovir in breast milk after valacyclovir administration is considerably less than that used in therapeutic dosing of neonates. The relative infant dose would be 4.7% of the maternal dose. See acyclovir.

Relative infant dose: 4.7%
Time to clear: Between 10 and 15 hours
Lactation risk category: L1
Pregnancy risk category: B
Adult dose: 500-1000 milligrams two to three times daily

Alternatives: Acyclovir

VALERIAN OFFICINALIS

Common names: Valerian Root
AAP recommendation: Not reviewed

Valerian root is most commonly used as a sedative/hypnotic. Of the numerous chemicals present in the root, the most important chemical group appears to be the valepotriates (sedatives). There are no reports on the transfer of valerian root compounds into breastmilk. However, the use of sedatives in breastfeeding mothers is generally discouraged due to a possible increased risk of sleep apnea and SIDS.

Relative infant dose:
Time to clear:
Lactation risk category: L3
Pregnancy risk category:
Adult dose:
Alternatives:

VALGANCICLOVIR

Trade names: Valcyte, Cytovene
AAP recommendation: Not reviewed

Valganciclovir is an inactive drug that is rapidly metabolized to the active antiviral drug, ganciclovir. It is used for cytomegalovirus infections particularly in HIV infected patients. There are no reports on its use in breastfeeding mothers, but oral absorption in the infant is likely low.

Relative infant dose:
Time to clear: Between 16 and 20 hours
Lactation risk category: L3
Pregnancy risk category: C
Adult dose: 450-900 milligrams daily
Alternatives:

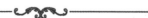

VALPROIC ACID

Trade names: Depakene, Depakote, Novo-Valproic, Deproic, Epilim, Valpro, Convulex

AAP recommendation: Maternal medication usually compatible with breastfeeding

Valproic acid is a popular anticonvulsant used in the management of seizures. Most authors of reported studies agree that the amount of valproic acid transferring to the infant via breastmilk is low. Breastfeeding would appear safe. Young women should probably be supplemented with folic acid.

Relative infant dose: 0.7%
Time to clear: Between 2.5 and 3 days
Lactation risk category: L2
Pregnancy risk category: D
Adult dose: 10-30 milligrams per kilogram daily
Alternatives:

VALSARTAN

Trade names: Diovan

AAP recommendation: Not reviewed

Valsartan is used to treat high blood pressure. There are no reports on the transfer of valsartan into breastmilk. Use with caution in pregnant mothers and in breastfeeding mothers with premature infants.

Relative infant dose:
Time to clear: Between 1.5 and 2 days
Lactation risk category: L4
Pregnancy risk category: D
Adult dose: 80-320 milligrams daily
Alternatives:

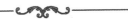

VANCOMYCIN

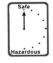

Trade names: Vancocin, Vancoled

AAP recommendation: Not reviewed

Vancomycin is an antibiotic commonly used in newborns and infants. Only low levels of vancomycin are secreted into breastmilk. Its poor absorption from the intestinal tract (less than 3%) would limit its absorption. Low levels in the infant could alter the gastrointestinal flora, but this is of minimal concern.

Relative infant dose: 6.7%
Time to clear: Between 22.5 and 28 hours
Lactation risk category: L1
Pregnancy risk category: C
Adult dose: 125-500 milligrams every 6 hours
Alternatives:

VARICELLA-ZOSTER VIRUS

Common names: Chickenpox
AAP recommendation: Not reviewed

Varicella-zoster virus (VZV) is the chickenpox virus. It is controversial whether the chickenpox virus will transfer to the infant through breastfeeding. In one study, it was reported that a mother transferred the virus to her breastfeeding infant. In two other studies, the virus could not be isolated in the breastmilk of the study participants. According to the American Academy of Pediatrics, neonates born to mothers with active varicella should be placed in isolation at birth and, if still hospitalized, until 21 or 28 days of age, depending on whether they received VZIG (Varicella Zoster Immune Globulin). Candidates for VZIG include: immunocompromised children, pregnant women, and a newborn infant whose mother has onset of VZV within 5 days before or 48 hours after delivery.

Relative infant dose:
Time to clear:
Lactation risk category: L4
Pregnancy risk category:
Adult dose:
Alternatives:

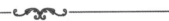

VASOPRESSIN

Trade names: Pitressin, Pressyn, Pitresin
AAP recommendation: Not reviewed

Vasopressin, also known as the antidiuretic hormone, reduces urine production by the kidney. Although it probably passes to some degree into breastmilk, it is rapidly destroyed in the gastrointestinal tract and must be administered by injection or intranasally. Oral absorption by a breastfeeding infant is very unlikely. A similar drug, demospressin, transfers into milk in extraordinarily low levels.

Relative infant dose:
Time to clear: Between 40 minutes and 1.5 hours
Lactation risk category: L3
Pregnancy risk category: B
Adult dose: 5-10 units two to four times daily as needed
Alternatives:

VENLAFAXINE

Trade names: Effexor, Efexor

AAP recommendation: Not reviewed

Venlafaxine is an antidepressant that is similar in mechanism to other antidepressants such as Prozac. Venlafaxine is transferred into breastmilk at moderate levels. The infant exposure to venlafaxine and its metabolite, O-desmethylvenlafaxine, is 6.4% of the maternal dose. The study reported that the infants were healthy and showed no acute harmful effects.

Relative infant dose: 6.4%
Time to clear: Between 20 and 25 hours
Lactation risk category: L3
Pregnancy risk category: C
Adult dose: 75 milligrams three times daily
Alternatives: Sertraline, Paroxetine

VERAPAMIL

Trade names: Calan, Isoptin, Covera-HS, Novo-Veramil,
                Anpec, Coridlox, Veracaps SR, Berkatens, Univer

AAP recommendation: Maternal medication usually compatible with
                        breastfeeding

Verapamil is used to lower high blood pressure. It is secreted into breastmilk at very low levels. The levels vary according to several studies. The relative infant dose can vary between 0.15 to 0.98% of the maternal dose. Regardless of the variability, the percent of the mother's dose that transfers to the infant is still quite small. See bepridil, diltiazem, nifedipine as alternates.

Relative infant dose: 1.0%
Time to clear: Between 12 hours and 1.5 days
Lactation risk category: L2
Pregnancy risk category: C
Adult dose: 80-100 milligrams three times daily
Alternatives: Bepridil, Nifedipine, Nimodipine

VIGABATRIN

Trade names: Sabril

AAP recommendation: Not reviewed

Vigabatrin is a newer anticonvulsant. Vigabatrin is an effective anticonvulsant for the treatment of multi-drug resistant complex partial seizures. There are no reports on the transfer of vigabatrin into breastmilk. Some caution is recommended in breastfeeding mothers.

Relative infant dose:
Time to clear: Between 1 and 1.5 days
Lactation risk category: L3
Pregnancy risk category:
Adult dose: 1-4 grams daily
Alternatives:

VITAMIN A

Trade names: Aquasol A, Del-VI-A, Vitamin A, Retinol, Avoleum

AAP recommendation: Not reviewed

Vitamin A (retinol) is a typical retinoid. It is a fat soluble vitamin that is secreted into breastmilk and mainly captured in high concentrations in the liver (90%). Retinol is absorbed in the small intestine. Levels in infants are generally unknown. The overdose of Vitamin A is extremely dangerous. Adults should never exceed 5000 units per day chronically. DO NOT use doses in breastfeeding mothers that are greater than 5000 units per day. Mature breastmilk is rich in retinol and contains 750 micrograms per liter (2800 units). Infants do not generally require vitamin A supplementation.

Relative infant dose:

Time to clear:
Lactation risk category: L3
Pregnancy risk category: A
Adult dose: < 5000 IU (international units) daily
Alternatives:

VITAMIN B-12

Trade names: Cyanocobalamin, Anacobin, Cytacon
AAP recommendation: Maternal medication usually compatible with
                                             breastfeeding

Vitamin B-12 is also called cyanocobalamin and is used for the treatment of anemia (chronic illness due to impaired vitamin B-12 absorption). It is an essential vitamin that is secreted into breastmilk. Vitamin B-12 deficiency is very dangerous to an infant. Milk levels vary in proportion to maternal serum levels. Vegetarian mothers may have low levels unless supplemented. Supplementation of breastfeeding mothers is generally recommended.

Relative infant dose:
Time to clear:
Lactation risk category: L1
Pregnancy risk category: A
Adult dose: 25 micrograms daily
Alternatives:

VITAMIN D

Trade names: Calciferol, Delta-D, Vitamin D, Calcijex,
                             Drisdol, Hytakerol, Radiostol
AAP recommendation: Maternal medication usually compatible with
                                             breastfeeding

Vitamin D is secreted into breastmilk in limited concentrations and is somewhat proportional to maternal serum levels. There is some concern that mothers deficient in vitamin D may not provide sufficient vitamin D to their infant. This may slow bone mineralization in their infants. Breastmilk is known to have low concentrations of vitamin D. On average, breast milk contains approximately 26 IU per liter (range = 5-136).

Supplementing a mother with even moderate doses of vitamin D does not substantially increase milk levels unless plasma levels are quite low. However, supplementing with high therapeutic doses (more than 5000 IU per day) for various syndromes can significantly elevate milk concentrations of vitamin D leading to potential hypercalcemia in a breastfed infant. Excessively high therapeutic doses should be used with great caution in a breastfeeding mother. Lower doses are suggested in undernourished mothers (RDA is 400-600 IU per day). In 2003, the Academy of Pediatrics, responding to the increased reports of rickets in breastfeeding infants, published a recommendation that all US infants should consume at least 200 IU of vitamin D per day by supplementation if needed.

These recommendations are somewhat controversial for at least two reasons. One, we do not know with certainty the minimal but adequate dose of vitamin D required by breastfed infants. Two, they suggest that a mother's milk may in some cases be nutritionally inadequate. Regardless of these concerns, mothers who have limited vitamin D intake due to poor nutrition or whose bodies have limited exposure to sunlight (northern climates), probably need supplementation as their milk is likely to be deficient in vitamin D. In addition, infants of these mothers who have limited or no exposure to sunlight or inadequate intake may need supplementation, as these infants (particularly dark skinned) are most at risk for developing rickets.

Relative infant dose:
Time to clear:
Lactation risk category: L3
Pregnancy risk category: A
Adult dose: 250 micrograms to 1.5 milligrams daily
Alternatives:

VITAMIN E

Trade names: Alpha Tocopherol, Aquasol E, Bio E
AAP recommendation: Not reviewed

Vitamin E (alpha tocopherol) is readily transferred into breastmilk. The recommended daily allowance (RDA) in breastfeeding mothers is approximately 16 IU per day. Using 50-100 IU per day would not be overly excessive. Do not use exceptionally high doses (1000 IU per day). Do not apply concentrated vitamin E to nipples.

Relative infant dose:
Time to clear: Between 47 and 59 days
Lactation risk category: L2
Pregnancy risk category: A
Adult dose: 16-18 international units (1 milligram d-A-tocopherol) daily

Alternatives:

WARFARIN

Trade names: Coumadin, Panwarfin, Warfilone, Marevan

AAP recommendation: Maternal medication usually compatible with breastfeeding

Warfarin is a potent anticoagulant (an agent that prevents blood from clotting). The transfer of warfarin into human milk is minimal. The amount depends to some degree on the dose administered. According to the authors of several published studies, maternal warfarin apparently poses little risk to a nursing infant and so far has not produced bleeding anomalies in breastfed infants. Other anticoagulants, such as phenindione, should be avoided. Observe infant for bleeding such as excessive bruising or reddish petechia (spots). While the risks in premature infants who are breastfed is still low, oral supplementation of the infant with vitamin K1 will preclude any chance of hemorrhage (bleeding). Even modest doses of Vitamin K counteract high doses of warfarin.

Relative infant dose:
Time to clear: Between 4 and 12.5 days
Lactation risk category: L2
Pregnancy risk category: D
Adult dose: 2-10 milligrams daily
Alternatives:

WEST NILE FEVER

Trade names:
AAP recommendation: Not reviewed

West Nile fever in humans is usually an influenza-like illness characterized by an abrupt onset (incubation period is 3 to 6 days) of moderate to high fever, sometimes with chills, headache (often frontal), sore throat, backache, muscle pain, bone pain, fatigue, reddening of the eyes, rash, loss of appetite, nausea, abdominal pain, diarrhea, and respiratory symptoms. It is not known whether the virus transfers into breastmilk or if it is communicable if present in milk. However, its transmission to a breastfed infant is believed unlikely. There have been no reports of a mother passing the West Nile virus via breastmilk to her infant.

Infected mosquitoes are the primary carrier for West Nile virus. Both hard and soft ticks have been found infected with West Nile virus in nature, but their role in the transmission and maintenance of the virus is uncertain. For answers to questions about West Nile virus, please see the CDC web site: http://www.cdc.gov/ncidod/dvbid/westnile/q&a.htm

Relative infant dose:
Time to clear:
Lactation risk category:
Pregnancy risk category:
Adult dose:
Alternatives:

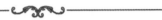

ZAFIRLUKAST

Trade names: Accolate

AAP recommendation: Not reviewed

Zafirlukast is used to prevent and treat asthma. Zafirlukast is not a bronchodilator and should not be used for acute asthma attacks. It is transferred into breastmilk in low concentrations and poorly absorbed when administered with food. It is likely the oral absorption via ingestion of breastmilk would be low.

Relative infant dose: 0.7%
Time to clear: Between 1.5 and 2.5 days
Lactation risk category: L3
Pregnancy risk category: B
Adult dose: 20 milligrams twice daily
Alternatives:

ZALEPLON

Trade names: Sonata

AAP recommendation: Not reviewed

Zaleplon is a hypnotic sedative. Zaleplon is transferred into breastmilk, but the authors of one study suggest that the infant would receive only small subclinical amounts.

Relative infant dose: 1.5%
Time to clear: Between 5 and 6 hours
Lactation risk category: L2
Pregnancy risk category: C

Adult dose: 10 milligrams nightly
Alternatives:

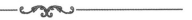

ZANAMIVIR

Trade names: Relenza
AAP recommendation: Not reviewed

Zanamivir is used in the treatment of acute illness caused by the influenza virus in adults and children younger than 7 years of age. It is only moderately effective and is believed to reduce symptoms by only 30% or several days, and only if treatment is instituted within 2 days of infection. It is administered via inhalation using a diskhaler device. Only 4-17% of the inhaled drug is systemically absorbed. There are no reports on the transfer of zanamivir into breastmilk. Due to the poor oral or inhaled absorption and the incredibly low plasma levels, it is unlikely to transfer into milk in relevant amounts or produce harmful effects in breastfed infants.

However, due to its limited effectiveness (reduces length of illness by 1 to 1.5 days), its use in breastfeeding mothers is probably not warranted unless in high-risk patients with other severe medical conditions.

Relative infant dose:
Time to clear: Between 10 and 25.5 hours
Lactation risk category: L3
Pregnancy risk category: B
Adult dose: 10 milligrams twice daily
Alternatives:

ZINC SALTS

Common names: Zinc
AAP recommendation: Not reviewed

Zinc is an essential element that is required for enzymatic function within the cell. Zinc deficiencies have been documented in newborns and premature infants with symptoms such as anorexia, arthritis, diarrheas, eczema (inflammation of the skin), recurrent infections and recalcitrant skin problems. The recommended daily allowance (RDA) for adults is 12-15 milligrams per day. The average oral dose of supplements is 25-50 milligrams per day. Higher doses may lead to gastritis, therefore excessive intake is detrimental. Interestingly, the oral absorption of dietary zinc is nearly twice as high in mothers during lactation as before conception.

There was no difference in serum zinc values between women who took iron supplements and those who did not; although, iron supplementation may reduce oral zinc absorption. Zinc absorption by the infant from breastmilk is high, averaging 41%. This is significantly higher than from soy or cow formulas (14% and 31% respectively). Minimum daily requirements of zinc in full term infants vary from 0.3 to 0.5 milligrams per kilogram per day.

Supplementation with 25-50 milligrams per day is probably safe, but excessive doses are discouraged. Another author has shown that zinc levels in breastmilk are independent of maternal plasma zinc concentrations or dietary zinc intake. Other body pools of zinc (ie, liver and bone) are perhaps the source of zinc in breastmilk. Therefore, higher levels of oral zinc intake probably have minimal effect on zinc concentrations in milk, but excessive doses are not recommended.

Relative infant dose:
Time to clear:
Lactation risk category: L2
Pregnancy risk category:
Adult dose: 15 milligrams daily
Alternatives:

ZOLMITRIPTAN

Trade names: Zomig, Zomig-ZMT, Rapimelt
AAP recommendation: Not reviewed

Zolmitriptan is used to treat acute migraine headaches. Zolmitriptan is structurally similar to sumatriptan but has better oral absorption, higher penetration into the central nervous system, and may have dual mechanisms of action. There are no reports on the transfer of zolmitriptan into breastmilk. See sumatriptan as a preferred alternate.

Relative infant dose:
Time to clear: Between 12 and 15 hours
Lactation risk category: L3
Pregnancy risk category: C
Adult dose: 2.5 milligrams every 2 hours as needed
Alternatives: Sumatriptan

ZOLPIDEM TARTRATE

Trade names: Ambien

AAP recommendation: Maternal medication usually compatible with breastfeeding

Zolpidem is used for the short-term treatment of insomnia (sleeplessness), although it is not part of the "Valium" family of drugs. The authors in one study suggest that the amount of zolpidem recovered in breastmilk 3 hours after administration ranged from 0.004 to 0.019% of the total maternal dose. Breastmilk clearance of zolpidem is very rapid and none was detectable (below 0.5 nanograms per milliliter) by 4-5 hours postdose. However, one case of infant sedation and poor appetite related to zolpidem use has been reported following the nightly use of sertraline (100 milligrams) and 10 milligrams Zolpidem. Upon discontinuation of zolpidem, the infant regained appetite and became more alert.

Relative infant dose:
Time to clear: Between 10 and 25 hours
Lactation risk category: L3
Pregnancy risk category: B
Adult dose: 5-10 milligrams daily
Alternatives:

ZONISAMIDE

Trade names: Zonegran

AAP recommendation: Not reviewed

Zonisamide is used in the treatment of seizures in children and epilepsy in adults. Using the highest reported breastmilk levels of zonisamide, the relative infant dose would be 33% of the maternal dose, which is quite high. Significant caution is recommended with this drug as a number of pediatric harmful effects have been noted in older children.

Relative infant dose: 33.3%
Time to clear: Between 10.5 and 13 days
Lactation risk category: L5
Pregnancy risk category: C
Adult dose: 100-200 milligrams per day
Alternatives:

ZOPICLONE

Trade names: Dom-Zopiclone, PMS-Zopiclone, Rhovan,
                 Alti-Zopiclone, Ratio-Zopiclone, Imovane, Zileze

AAP recommendation: Not reviewed

Zopiclone is a sedative/hypnotic which, although structurally dissimilar to the "Valium family", has the same effect. The authors report that the average infant dose of Zopiclone via breastmilk would be 1.4% of the maternal dose.

Relative infant dose: 1.5%
Time to clear: Between 16 and 25 hours
Lactation risk category: L2
Pregnancy risk category:
Adult dose: 7.5 milligrams by mouth
Alternatives:

Appendix

Normal growth during development*

BOYS	Weight (lb.)	Length (in.)	Head circumference (in.)
Birth	7.5	19.9	13.9
3 months	12.6	23.8	16.1
6 months	16.7	26.1	17.3
9 months	20.0	28	18.1
12 months	22.2	29.6	18.6
15 months	23.7	30.9	18.9
18 months	25.2	32.2	19.2
24 months	27.7	34.4	19.6

GIRLS	Weight (lb.)	Length (in.)	Head circumference (in.)
Birth	7.2	19.7	13.5
3 months	11.8	23.5	15.6
6 months	15.9	25.8	16.7
9 months	18.8	27.7	17.4
12 months	21.0	29.3	17.9
15 months	22.5	30.6	18.4
18 months	23.9	31.9	18.6
24 months	26.3	34.0	18.8

* Please note: these data were not derived from exclusively breastfed infants.

Recommended childhood and adolescent immunization schedule – United States 2005

Age \ Vaccine	Birth	1 mo	2 mo	4 mo	6 mo	12 mo	15 mo	18 mo	24 mo	4 – 6 yrs	11 – 12 yrs	13 – 18 yrs
DTP			DTP	DTP	DTP		DTP	DTP		DTP	Td	Td
Hib			Hib	Hib	Hib	Hib	Hib					
Hepatitis A										Hepatitis A series*		
Hepatitis B	HB#1	HB#1 / HB #2	HB #2			HB #3	HB #3				HB series	
Inactivated Poliovirus			IPV	IPV		IPV	IPV			IPV		
Influenza						Ifz yearly	Ifz yearly			Ifz yearly		
MMR						MMR #1	MMR #1			MMR #2	MMR #2	
Pneumococcal			PCV	PCV	PCV	PCV	PCV		PCV	PPV		
Varicella						Varicella	Varicella			Varicella	Varicella	

DTP = Diphtheria, Tetanus, Pertussis; Hib = *Haemophilus influenzae* type b; HB = Hepatitis B; IPV = Inactivated poliovirus; Ifz = influenza; MMR = Measles, Mumps & Rubella; PCV = Pneumococcal conjugate vaccine; PPV = Pneumococcal polysaccharide vaccine; Td = Tetanus & Diphtheria
◻ = range of recommended age; ▨ = catch-up immunization; ▨ = preadolescent assessment; ▨ = the first Hepatitis B dose can be given at 1 or 2 months of age only if the mother tests negative for hepatitis B surface antigen (HBsAg); * = Hep A is recommended for adults and children in selected states, regions and for people in a high risk category. Note that there need to be at least a 6 month period between the two doses. Contact the public health authority near you.

Vaccines

Vaccine	Information for breastfeeding mothers
Anthrax	• No data available in breastfeeding women, although it is unlikely to transfer into breastmilk. • Not "medically contraindicated" by the CDC[1] for breastfeeding women. • Not for use by pregnant women.
Cholera	• Not contraindicated for breastfeeding women.
Diphtheria and tetanus toxoid	• The CDC[1] suggests that there are no risks for the infant associated with its use in breastfeeding mothers.
Diphtheria-Tetanus-Pertussis (DTP)	• Pertussis vaccines are generally contraindicated for people over the age of 7 and therefore it is not indicated for use in mothers. • However, there is no specific contraindication in breastfeeding women.
Haemophilus B conjugate vaccine	• No contraindication although it is not indicated for use in adults.
Hepatitis A	• Although no data are available on its use in breastfeeding women, it can be used in pregnant women after 14 weeks and in children 2 years of age. • The CDC[1] recommends considering the immune globulin rather than the vaccine.
Hepatitis B	• Commonly used in breastfeeding mothers and even their infants. Safe.
Influenza	• Commonly used in breastfeeding mothers. Use the inactivated vaccine if possible.
Lyme Disease Vaccine	• It is primarily indicated for individuals 15-70 years of age. • The CDC[1] suggests it can be used in breastfeeding patients.

Vaccine	Information for breastfeeding mothers
Meningococcal	• There are no contraindications for its use in breastfeeding mothers other than allergic hypersensitivity to some of the ingredients. Safe for breastfeeding mothers.
Measles, Mumps and Rubella (MMR)	• If medically required, MMR vaccine can be administered early postpartum to breastfeeding mothers. • CONTRAINDICATED in pregnant women.
Polio	• Wait until infant is 6 weeks of age before immunizing breastfeeding mother, but it would not harm a breastfeeding infant.
Rabies	• Although no data are available on its transfer into breastmilk, it is unlikely to produce untoward effects in breastfed infants.
Rubella	• The CDC[1] recommends the early postpartum immunization of women who show no or low antibody titers to rubella. • In general, the use of rubella virus vaccine in mothers of full-term normal infants has not been associated with untoward effects and is generally recommended.
Smallpox	• No data are available suggesting the degree of transmission into breastmilk, but it is likely to enter breastmilk to some degree. • According to the CDC[1], the use of smallpox vaccinations is not justified in breastfeeding mothers who are not at high risk.
Typhoid	• No data are available on its transfer into breastmilk but it is unlikely. • If immunization is required, the injectable vaccine as opposed to the oral dosage form would be preferred, as infection of the neonate would be possible from the latter.

Vaccine	Information for breastfeeding mothers
Varicella	• Mothers of infants with weak immune systems should not breastfeed following use of this vaccine. • Both the AAP[2] and the CDC[1] approved the use of Varicella-Zoster vaccines in breastfeeding mothers if the risk of infection is high.
Yellow fever	• There is a possible risk that the weakened virus can transfer into breastmilk. • Whenever possible, vaccination of a nursing mother should be avoided. • However, the CDC[1] and ACIP[3] recommend that nursing mothers receive the vaccine **if travel into areas of high yellow fever risk** cannot be postponed. • Only given to pregnant women if clearly needed if travel into high risk areas cannot be postponed and then during the second and third trimester to minimize concern over birth defects. The infant should be closely monitored.

[1] CDC = Center for Disease Control and Prevention;
[2] AAP = American Academy of Pediatrics;
[3] ACIP = Advisory Committee on Immunization Practices

Drugs that are usually not to be used in lactating women[1]

Drug	Nature of possible risk to infant
Amiodarone	Relative infant dose 43% of maternal dose; may accumulate because of very long half-life; adverse cardiovascular and thyroid effects possible.
Antineoplastic agents	Overtly toxic; avoid exposure; bone marrow suppression, damage to intestinal epithelial cells possible.
Chloramphenicol	Relative infant dose 2% of maternal dose. Blood dyscrasias, aplastic anemia, etc. is possible.
Ergotamine	Symptoms of ergotism (vomiting and diarrhea) reported; potential to inhibit prolactin secretion.
Gold salts	Relative infant dose varies from 1-7%. Long half-life in adults suggests potential for accumulation. Possibility of diarrhea, dermatitis, nephrotoxicity and blood dyscrasias.
Lithium	Not recommended or use great caution in breastfeeding mothers. Infant plasma levels may approach 30-40% of maternal plasma levels.
Phenindione	Relative infant dose calculated at around 18% of maternal dose and abnormal blood coagulation in an infant has been reported.
Pseudoephedrine	New data suggest that pseudoephedrine may inhibit prolactin and milk production significantly in some mothers.

Drug	Nature of possible risk to infant
Radiopharmaceuticals	Temporary discontinuation of breast-feeding may be necessary. See the Nuclear Regulatory Commission (NRC) table on this website: http://neonatal.ama.ttuhsc.edu/lact/
Retinoids	• Oral retinoids (e.g. isotretinoin) should not be used due to the higher risk to the infant and likely distribution to milk. • Topical retinoids (e.g. tretinoin) are probably safe to use on moderate to small surface areas of the body.
Tetracyclines (Chronic)	While the acute use of tetracyclines for up to 3 weeks is okay, chronic use over many months may lead to staining of immature teeth, or changes in epiphyseal bone growth.

[1] Adapted from Hale TW, Ilett KF. Drug Therapy and Breastfeeding: From Theory to Clinical Practice, First Edition ed. London: Parthenon Publishing; 2002

Can I breastfeed if I have …?

(Please refer to the individual monographs if you are using
medication for the listed condition/disease)

Condition/ disease	Information for breastfeeding mothers
Asthma	Medications used for asthma are in general compatible with breastfeeding.
Atopic dermatitis (eczema)	Mothers with eczema can breastfeed.
Cancer	• Breastfeeding can generally continue during the assessment period if maternal cancer is suspected during lactation and when the mother receives external or localized radiation therapy. • In the case of breast cancer where the mother receives radiation directly to the breast, breastfeeding can continue on the unaffected breast since radiation may affect milk production. "Pump-and-discard" after treatment is received, for a time period depending on the specific medication, after which breastfeeding can continue.
Candidiasis (Moniliasis/ yeast infection)	Breastfeeding can continue throughout episodes of infection of the nipples, vagina or mouth.
Chickenpox (Varicella Zoster virus)	It is controversial whether the chickenpox virus will transfer to the infant through breastfeeding. The infected mother and infant should be separated until all the mother's lesions are crusted over and until she is no longer infectious. The infant should receive anti-viral drugs and VZIG (Varicella Zoster Immune Globulin).
Common cold	Breastfeeding should be continued if the mother has a cold.

Condition/ disease	Information for breastfeeding mothers
Crohn's disease (regional enteritis)	It is recommended that breastfeeding continue if parents have a family history of Crohn's disease.
Cystic fibrosis	Breastfeeding is encouraged, with careful monitoring of the nutritional status and health of the nursing mother.
Diabetes mellitus	Refer to the individual monographs on the drugs used to treat diabetes mellitus. Breastfeeding is strongly encouraged.
Flu (influenza)	Although good hygiene is encouraged around the infant, breastfeeding can continue.
Galactoceles	Breastfeeding can continue.
German measles (Rubella)	Breastfeeding can continue.
Gonorrhea	Treatment should commence promptly. If an untreated infected mother gave birth, she and the infant (prophylactic) need to receive therapy. Breastfeeding can continue if treatment is initiated or imminent.
Strep throat	Breastfeeding can continue, but precautions need to be taken when handling the infant to avoid transmission.
Hepatitis A, B & C	Breastfeeding can continue.
Herpes simplex	Breastfeeding can continue, unless the nipple or areola has active lesions in which case breastfeeding on the affected breast should be postponed until the breast has healed. Lesions on other areas of the breast need to be covered when breastfeeding.

Condition/ disease	Information for breastfeeding mothers
HIV	The World Health Organization (WHO) recommends that exclusive breastfeeding continue for a period of 6 months irrespective of HIV status in nations where malnutrition and infectious diseases create a high infant mortality risk. However, in nations where safe alternative feeding methods are available, nursing is contraindicated.
Mastitis	Breastfeeding should continue since interrupting breastfeeding may cause engorgement and possibly abscess formation. A clinician should evaluate the nursing mother.
Menstrual cramps	Breastfeeding can continue in women with primary dysmenorrheal (menstrual cramps).
Postpartum depression	Postpartum depression is dangerous to the infant's psychological development and must be treated. There are numerous antidepressant medications that are suitable for breastfeeding mothers. Breastfeeding should continue.
Psoriasis	Although the specific medication might pose concern, mothers with psoriasis can breastfeed.
Rabies	When encountering a rabies source, a nursing mother should initiate vaccination and receive the human rabies immune globulin. Breastfeeding may subsequently continue.
Rubella	Breastfeeding can continue.
Sheehan's syndrome	Lactation failure is possible in patients with Sheehan's syndrome.
Sickle cell disease	Breastfeeding can continue.
Syphilis	When treatment is initiated or imminent, an infected mother can breastfeed.
Toxoplasmosis	Breastfeeding can continue.

Condition/ disease	Information for breastfeeding mothers
Trichomoniasis	The nursing mother should "pump-and-discard" for 12 to 24 hours after receiving metronidazole single dose therapy (2 grams), after which breastfeeding can continue. Mothers that take lower doses per day can continue to breastfeed.
Ulcerative colitis	Breastfeeding can continue.
Urinary tract infection	Breastfeeding can continue.

Source: Merewood, A & Philipp, B.L. 2001. Breastfeeding conditions and diseases. 1st edition. Pharmasoft publishing. p. 267

Topical corticosteroids

Potency	Topical corticosteroid (Brand name)	Preparation	Comment
Low potency	Alclometasone (Aclovate)	0.05% cream/ ointment	Probably safe if not used in large amounts.
	Desonide (DesOwen, Tridesilon)	0.05% cream	
	Fluocinolone (Synalar solution, Derma-Smoothe/FS)	0.01% cream/ solution	
	Hydrocortisone (Anusol-HC, Cortaid, Cortizone, Dermarest, Hytone, ProctoCream)	0.25%; 0.5%; 1% & 2.5% in various dosage forms	
Intermediate potency	Betamethasone (Alphatrex, Betatrex)	0.025% cream/ gel/lotion 0.05% lotion 0.1% cream	Probably safe if used in minimal amounts directly applied on the nipple. Some caution is recommended.
	Clocortolone (Cloderm)	0.1% cream	
	Desoximetasone (Topicort-LP)	0.05% cream	
	Fluocinolone (Synalar)	0.025% cream/ ointment	
	Flurandrenolide (Cordran)	0.05% cream/ ointment/ lotion/tape	
	Fluticasone (Cutivate)	0.005% ointment & 0.05% cream	
	Hydrocortisone butyrate or valerate (Locoid, Locoid Lipocream, Westcort)	0.1% ointment/ solution & 0.2% cream/ ointment	
	Mometasone furoate (Elecon)	0.1% cream/ ointment/lotion	
	Prednicarbate (Dermatop)	0.1% cream/ ointment	
	Triamcinolone acetonide (Aristocort, Kenalog, Triderm)	0.025% & 0.1% cream/ ointment/lotion	

Potency	Topical corticosteroid (Brand name)	Preparation	Comment
High potency	Amcinonide (Cyclocort)	0.1% cream/ ointment/lotion	Do not use on nipple. Caution is recommended if used topically on large surface areas.
	Betamethasone dipropionate or valerate (Alphatrex, Betatrex, Diprolene AF, Diprolene, Maxivate)	0.05% cream/ ointment & 0.1% ointment	
	Desoximetasone (Topicort)	0.05% gel & 0.25% cream/ ointment	
	Diflorasone diacetate (Maxiflor, Psorcon)	0.05% cream/ ointment	
	Fluocinonide (Lidex, Lidex-E)	0.05% cream/ ointment/gel	
	Halcinonide (Halog, Halog-E)	0.1% cream/ ointment	
	Triamcinolone (Aristocort, Kenalog)	0.5% cream/ ointment	
Very high potency	Clobetasol (Clobex, Cormax, Olux, Temovate)	0.05% cream/ ointment /lotion/foam	Never use on nipple. Caution is recommended if used topically on large surface areas.
	Diflorasone diacetate (Maxiflor, Psorcon)	0.05% ointment	
	Halobetasol (Ultravate)	0.05% cream/ ointment	

Is it a cold or the flu?

Symptoms	Cold	Flu
fever	rare	characteristic, high (102-104F); lasts 3-4 days
headache	rare	prominent
general aches, pains	slight	usual; often severe
fatigue, weakness	quite mild	can last up to 2-3 weeks
extreme exhaustion	never	early and prominent
stuffy nose	common	sometimes
sneezing	usual	sometimes
sore throat	common	sometimes
chest discomfort, cough	mild to moderate; hacking cough	common; can become severe

Source: National Institute of Allergy and Infectious Diseases
Publication No. (FDA) 99-1264
http://www.fda.gov/fdac/features/896_flu.html

Cold Remedies

Trade Name	Ingredients	Comments
666 cold preparation, maximum strength liquid	Acetaminophen, Pseudoephedrine, Dextromethorphan	Probably safe but may suppress milk supply.
Actifed cold & allergy tablets	Triprolidine, Pseudoephedrine	Probably safe; observe for sedation and may suppress milk supply.
Actifed cold & sinus maximum strength tablets	Acetaminophen, Chlorpheniramine, Pseudoephedrine	Probably safe; observe for sedation and may suppress milk supply.
Advil allergy sinus tablets	Chlorpheniramine, Ibuprofen, Pseudoephedrine	Probably safe; observe for sedation and may suppress milk supply.
Advil cold & sinus liqui-gels	Ibuprofen, Pseudoephedrine	Probably safe but may suppress milk supply.
Advil cold & sinus tablets	Ibuprofen, Pseudoephedrine	Probably safe but may suppress milk supply.
Advil flu & body ache tablets	Ibuprofen, Pseudoephedrine	Probably safe but may suppress milk supply.
Alavert allergy & sinus D-12 hour tablets	Loratadine, Pseudoephedrine	Probably safe but may suppress milk supply.
Aleve cold & sinus tablets	Naproxen, Pseudoephedrine	Probably safe but may suppress milk supply.
Aleve sinus & headache tablets	Naproxen, Pseudoephedrine	Probably safe but may suppress milk supply.
Alka-Seltzer plus liqui-gels flu medicine	Acetaminophen, Pseudoephedrine, Dextromethorphan	Probably safe but may suppress milk supply.
Alka-Seltzer plus cold & cough liqui-gels	Acetaminophen, Chlorpheniramine, Dextromethorphan, Pseudoephedrine	Probably safe; observe for sedation, may suppress milk supply.
Alka-Seltzer plus cold & cough medicine effervescent tablets	Chlorpheniramine, Phenylephrine, Dextromethorphan	Probably safe; observe for sedation.
Alka-Seltzer plus cold & flu liqui-gels	Acetaminophen, Pseudoephedrine, Dextromethorphan	Probably safe but may suppress milk supply.

Trade Name	Ingredients	Comments
Alka-Seltzer plus cold & sinus liqui-gels	Acetaminophen, Pseudoephedrine	Probably safe but may suppress milk supply.
Alka-Seltzer plus cold & sinus tablets	Acetaminophen Phenylephrine	Probably safe
Alka-Seltzer plus cold medicine liqui-gels	Acetaminophen, Chlorpheniramine, Pseudoephedrine	Probably safe; observe for sedation and may suppress milk supply.
Alka-Seltzer plus cold medicine effervescent tablets	Acetaminophen, Chlorpheniramine, Phenylephrine	Probably safe; observe for sedation.
Alka-Seltzer plus flu medicine effervescent tablets	Aspirin, Chlorpheniramine, Dextromethorphan	Probably safe; observe for sedation.
Alka-Seltzer plus nightTime cold liqui-gels	Acetaminophen, Doxylamine, Pseudoephedrine, Dextromethorphan	Probably safe; observe for sedation and may suppress milk supply.
Alka-Seltzer plus night-time cold medicine effervescent	Doxylamine, Phenylephrine, Dextromethorphan	Probably safe; observe for sedation.
Alka-Seltzer plus nose & throat effervescent tablets	Acetaminophen, Chlorpheniramine, Dextromethorphan, Phenylephrine	Probably safe; observe for sedation.
Allegra-D tablets	Fexofenadine, Pseudoephedrine	Probably safe but may suppress milk supply.
Allerest allergy & sinus relief maximum strength tablets	Acetaminophen, Pseudoephedrine	Probably safe but may suppress milk supply.
Allerest maximum strength tablets	Chlorpheniramine, Pseudoephedrine	Probably safe; observe for sedation and may suppress milk supply.
Aprodine tablets	Triprolidine, Pseudoephedrine	Probably safe; observe for sedation and may suppress milk supply.
Benadryl allergy & cold tablets	Acetaminophen, Diphenhydramine, Pseudoephedrine	Probably safe; observe for sedation and may suppress milk supply.

Trade Name	Ingredients	Comments
Benadryl allergy & sinus fastmelt dissolving tablets	Diphenhydramine Pseudoephedrine	Probably safe; observe for sedation and may suppress milk supply.
Benadryl allergy & sinus headache tablets	Acetaminophen, Diphenhydramine, Pseudoephedrine	Probably safe; observe for sedation and may suppress milk supply.
Benadryl allergy & sinus liquid	Diphenhydramine, Pseudoephedrine	Probably safe; observe for sedation and may suppress milk supply.
Benadryl allergy & sinus tablets	Diphenhydramine, Pseudoephedrine	Probably safe; observe for sedation and may suppress milk supply.
Benadryl maximum strength severe allergy & sinus headache tablets	Acetaminophen, Diphenhydramine, Pseudoephedrine	Probably safe; observe for sedation and may suppress milk supply.
Benylin expectorant liquid	Guaifenesin, Dextromethorphan	Probably safe
Bromfed capsules	Brompheniramine, Pseudoephedrine	Probably safe; observe for sedation and may suppress milk supply.
Bromfed syrup	Brompheniramine, Pseudoephedrine	Probably safe; observe for sedation and may suppress milk supply.
Bromfed tablets	Brompheniramine, Pseudoephedrine	Probably safe; observe for sedation and may suppress milk supply.
Cardec DM syrup	Carbinoxamine, Pseudoephedrine, Dextromethorphan	Probably safe; observe for sedation and may suppress milk supply.
Cepacol sore throat liquid	Acetaminophen, Pseudoephedrine	Probably safe but may suppress milk supply.
Cheracol cough syrup	Guaifenesin, Codeine	Probably safe; observe for sedation.
Cheracol D cough formula syrup	Guaifenesin, Dextromethorphan	Probably safe
Cheracol plus liquid	Guaifenesin, Dextromethorphan	Probably safe
Chlor-Trimeton allergy-D 12 hour tablets	Chlorpheniramine, Pseudoephedrine	Probably safe; observe for sedation and may suppress milk supply.
Chlor-Trimeton allergy-D 4 hour tablets	Chlorpheniramine, Pseudoephedrine	Probably safe; observe for sedation and may suppress milk supply.

Trade Name	Ingredients	Comments
Claritin-D 12 hour/ Claritin-D 24 hour tablets	Loratadine, Pseudoephedrine	Probably safe but may suppress milk supply.
Codiclear DH syrup	Guaifenesin, Hydrocodone	Probably safe; observe for sedation.
Codimal DH syrup	Pyrilamine, Phenylephrine, Hydrocodone	Probably safe; observe for sedation.
Codimal DM syrup	Pyrilamine, Phenylephrine, Dextromethorphan	Probably safe; observe for sedation.
Coldec D tablets	Carbinoxamine, Pseudoephedrine	Probably safe; observe for sedation and may suppress milk supply.
Coldmist LA tablets	Guaifenesin, Pseudoephedrine	Probably safe but may suppress milk supply.
Comtrex allergy-sinus treatment, maximum strength tablets	Acetaminophen, Chlorpheniramine, Pseudoephedrine	Probably safe; observe for sedation and may suppress milk supply.
Comtrex cough and cold relief, multi-symptom maximum strength tablets	Acetaminophen, Chlorpheniramine, Pseudoephedrine, Dextromethorphan	Probably safe; observe for sedation and may suppress milk supply.
Comtrex day & night cold & cough relief, multi-symptom maximum strength tablets	Acetaminophen, Chlorpheniramine, Pseudoephedrine, Dextromethorphan	Probably safe; observe for sedation and may suppress milk supply.
Comtrex flu therapy & fever relief day & night, multi-symptom maximum strength tablets	Acetaminophen, Chlorpheniramine, Pseudoephedrine	Probably safe; observe for sedation and may suppress milk supply.
Comtrex multi-symptom deep chest cold & congestion relief softgels	Acetaminophen, Guaifenesin, Pseudoephedrine, Dextromethorphan	Probably safe but may suppress milk supply.

Trade Name	Ingredients	Comments
Comtrex multi-symptom maximum strength non-drowsy cold & cough relief tablets	Acetaminophen, Pseudoephedrine, Dextromethorphan	Probably safe but may suppress milk supply.
Contac day & night allergy/ sinus relief tablets	Acetaminophen, Diphenhydramine, Pseudoephedrine	Probably safe; observe for sedation and may suppress milk supply.
Contac day & night cold & flu tablets	Acetaminophen, Diphenhydramine, Pseudoephedrine, Dextromethorphan	Probably safe; observe for sedation and may suppress milk supply.
Contac severe cold & flu maximum strength tablets	Acetaminophen, Chlorpheniramine, Pseudoephedrine, Dextromethorphan	Probably safe; observe for sedation and may suppress milk supply.
Coricidin 'D' cold, flu & sinus tablets	Acetaminophen, Chlorpheniramine, Pseudoephedrine	Probably safe; observe for sedation and may suppress milk supply.
Coricidin HBP cold & flu tablets	Acetaminophen, Chlorpheniramine	Probably safe; observe for sedation.
Coricidin HBP cough & cold tablets	Chlorpheniramine, Dextromethorphan	Probably safe; observe for sedation.
Coricidin HBP maximum strength flu tablets	Acetaminophen, Chlorpheniramine, Dextromethorphan	Probably safe; observe for sedation.
Deconamine SR capsules	Chlorpheniramine, Pseudoephedrine	Probably safe; observe for sedation and may suppress milk supply.
Deconamine syrup	Chlorpheniramine, Pseudoephedrine	Probably safe; observe for sedation and may suppress milk supply.
Deconamine tablets	Chlorpheniramine, Pseudoephedrine	Probably safe; observe for sedation and may suppress milk supply.
Dihistine DH elixir	Chlorpheniramine, Pseudoephedrine, Codeine	Probably safe; observe for sedation and may suppress milk supply.
Dimetane-DX cough	Brompheniramine, Pseudoephedrine, Dextromethorphan	Probably safe; observe for sedation and may suppress milk supply.

Trade Name	Ingredients	Comments
Dimetapp long acting cough plus cold syrup	Pseudoephedrine, Dextromethorphan	Probably safe but may suppress milk supply.
Dristan cold multi-symptom formula tablets	Acetaminophen, Chlorpheniramine, Phenylephrine	Probably safe; observe for sedation.
Dristan cold non-drowsy maximum strength tablets	Acetaminophen, Pseudoephedrine	Probably safe but may suppress milk supply.
Dristan sinus tablets	Ibuprofen, Pseudoephedrine	Probably safe but may suppress milk supply.
Drixoral allergy sinus tablets	Acetaminophen, Dexbrompheniramine, Pseudoephedrine	Probably safe; observe for sedation and may suppress milk supply.
Drixoral cold & allergy tablets	Dexbrompheniramine, Pseudoephedrine	Probably safe; observe for sedation and may suppress milk supply.
Duratuss GP tablets	Guaifenesin, Pseudoephedrine	Probably safe but may suppress milk supply.
Duratuss HD elixir	Guaifenesin, Pseudoephedrine, Hydrocodone	Probably safe; observe for sedation and may suppress milk supply.
Duratuss tablets	Guaifenesin, Pseudoephedrine	Probably safe but may suppress milk supply.
Dura-Vent/DA tablets	Chlorpheniramine, Phenylephrine, Methscopolamine	Probably safe; observe for sedation.
Duraxin capsules	Acetaminophen, Phenyltoloxamine, Salicylamide	Probably safe; observe for sedation.
Dynex tablets	Guaifenesin, Pseudoephedrine	Probably safe but may suppress milk supply.
Endal tablets / Endal Nasal Decongestant tablets	Guaifenesin, Phenylephrine	Probably safe
Entex HC liquid	Guaifenesin, Phenylephrine, Hydrocodone	Probably safe; observe for sedation.
Entex LA tablets/capsules	Guaifenesin, Phenylephrine	Probably safe
Entex liquid	Guaifenesin, Phenylephrine	Probably safe

Trade Name	Ingredients	Comments
Entex PSE tablets/capsules	Guaifenesin, Pseudoephedrine	Probably safe but may suppress milk supply.
Genac tablets	Triprolidine, Pseudoephedrine	Probably safe; observe for sedation and may suppress milk supply.
Guaifed capsules	Guaifenesin, Pseudoephedrine	Probably safe but may suppress milk supply.
Guaifed-PD capsules	Guaifenesin, Phenylephrine	Probably safe
Guaifenex PSE 120 tablets	Guaifenesin, Pseudoephedrine	Probably safe but may suppress milk supply.
Guaifenex-Rx tablets	Guaifenesin, Pseudoephedrine	Probably safe but may suppress milk supply.
Guiatuss PE liquid	Guaifenesin, Pseudoephedrine	Probably safe but may suppress milk supply.
Histex HC liquid	Carbinoxamine, Hydrocodone, Pseudoephedrine	Probably safe; observe for sedation and may suppress milk supply.
Histex liquid	Chlorpheniramine, Pseudoephedrine	Probably safe; observe for sedation and may suppress milk supply.
Histex SR capsules	Brompheniramine, Pseudoephedrine	Probably safe; observe for sedation and may suppress milk supply.
Histussin HC syrup	Chlorpheniramine, Phenylephrine, Hydrocodone	Probably safe; observe for sedation.
Hycodan syrup	Hydrocodone, Homatropine	Probably safe; observe for sedation.
Hycodan tablets	Hydrocodone, Homatropine	Probably safe; observe for sedation.
Levall 5.0 liquid	Guaifenesin, Phenylephrine, Hydrocodone	Probably safe; observe for sedation.
Levall liquid	Carbetapentane, Guaifenesin, Phenylephrine	Probably safe; observe for sedation.
Liquibid-PD/ Liquibid-D 1200 tablets	Guaifenesin, Phenylephrine	Probably safe
Lodrane liquid	Brompheniramine, Pseudoephedrine	Probably safe; observe for sedation and may suppress milk supply.

Trade Name	Ingredients	Comments
Maxifed DMX tablets	Guaifenesin, Pseudoephedrine, Dextromethorphan	Probably safe but may suppress milk supply.
Motrin sinus headache tablets	Ibuprofen, Pseudoephedrine	Probably safe but may suppress milk supply.
Naldecon senior DX liquid	Guaifenesin, Dextromethorphan	Probably safe
Nucofed expectorant syrup	Guaifenesin, Pseudoephedrine, Codeine	Probably safe; observe for sedation and may suppress milk supply.
Nucotuss expectorant syrup	Guaifenesin, Pseudoephedrine, Codeine	Probably safe; observe for sedation and may suppress milk supply.
OMNIhist LA tablets	Chlorpheniramine, Phenylephrine, Methscopolamine	Probably safe; observe for sedation.
PanMist JR tablets	Guaifenesin, Pseudoephedrine	Probably safe but may suppress milk supply.
PanMist LA tablets	Guaifenesin, Pseudoephedrine	Probably safe but may suppress milk supply.
PanMist-DM syrup	Guaifenesin, Pseudoephedrine, Dextromethorphan	Probably safe but may suppress milk supply.
PanMist-S syrup	Guaifenesin, Pseudoephedrine	Probably safe but may suppress milk supply.
Percogesic extra strength tablets	Acetaminophen, Diphenhydramine	Probably safe; observe for sedation.
Percogesic tablets	Acetaminophen, Phenyltoloxamine	Probably safe; observe for sedation.
Phenergan VC syrup	Promethazine, Phenylephrine	Caution; observe for sedation
Polaramine expectorant liquid	Dexchlorpheniramine, Guaifenesin, Pseudoephedrine	Probably safe; observe for sedation and may suppress milk supply.
Primatene tablets	Guaifenesin, Ephedrine	Unsafe
Prolex DH liquid	Hydrocodone, K Guaicolsulfonate	Probably safe; observe for sedation.
Prometh VC w/ codeine cough syrup	Promethazine, Phenylephrine, Codeine	Unsafe

Trade Name	Ingredients	Comments
Promethazine HCL with codeine syrup	Promethazine, Codeine	Unsafe
Rescon-GG liquid	Guaifenesin, Phenylephrine	Probably safe
Robitussin allergy & cough liquid	Brompheniramine, Pseudoephedrine, Dextromethorphan	Probably safe; observe for sedation and may suppress milk supply.
Robitussin CF syrup	Guaifenesin, Pseudoephedrine, Dextromethorphan	Probably safe but may suppress milk supply.
Robitussin cold sinus & congestion tablets	Acetaminophen, Guaifenesin, Pseudoephedrine	Probably safe but may suppress milk supply.
Robitussin cold, cold & congestion softgels & tablets	Guaifenesin, Pseudoephedrine, Dextromethorphan	Probably safe but may suppress milk supply.
Robitussin cold, cold & cough softgels	Guaifenesin, Pseudoephedrine, Dextromethorphan	Probably safe but may suppress milk supply.
Robitussin cold, multi-symptom cold & flu softgels	Acetaminophen, Guaifenesin, Pseudoephedrine, Dextromethorphan	Probably safe but may suppress milk supply.
Robitussin cold, multi-symptom cold & flu tablets	Acetaminophen, Guaifenesin, Pseudoephedrine, Dextromethorphan	Probably safe but may suppress milk supply.
Robitussin cough & congestion formula liquid	Guaifenesin, Dextromethorphan	Probably safe
Robitussin flu liquid	Acetaminophen, Chlorpheniramine, Pseudoephedrine, Dextromethorphan	Probably safe; observe for sedation and may suppress milk supply.
Robitussin honey cough & cold liquid	Pseudoephedrine, Dextromethorphan	Probably safe but may suppress milk supply.
Robitussin honey flu multi-symptom liquid	Acetaminophen, Pseudoephedrine, Dextromethorphan	Probably safe but may suppress milk supply.

Trade Name	Ingredients	Comments
Robitussin honey flu nighttime syrup	Acetaminophen, Chlorpheniramine, Pseudoephedrine, Dextromethorphan	Probably safe; observe for sedation and may suppress milk supply.
Robitussin honey flu non-drowsy syrup	Acetaminophen, Pseudoephedrine, Dextromethorphan	Probably safe but may suppress milk supply.
Robitussin maximum strength cough & cold syrup	Pseudoephedrine, Dextromethorphan	Probably safe but may suppress milk supply.
Robitussin night relief liquid	Acetaminophen, Pyrilamine, Pseudoephedrine, Dextromethorphan	Probably safe; observe for sedation and may suppress milk supply.
Robitussin PE liquid	Guaifenesin, Pseudoephedrine	Probably safe but may suppress milk supply.
Robitussin severe congestion liqui-gels	Guaifenesin, Pseudoephedrine	Probably safe but may suppress milk supply.
Robitussin sugar free cough liquid	Guaifenesin, Dextromethorphan	Probably safe
Robitussin-DM liquid	Guaifenesin, Dextromethorphan	Probably safe
Rondec syrup	Brompheniramine, Pseudoephedrine	Probably safe; observe for sedation and may suppress milk supply.
Rondec tablets	Carbinoxamine, Pseudoephedrine	Probably safe; observe for sedation and may suppress milk supply.
Rondec-DM syrup	Brompheniramine, Pseudoephedrine, Dextromethorphan	Probably safe; observe for sedation and may suppress milk supply.
Rondec-TR tablets	Carbinoxamine, Pseudoephedrine	Probably safe; observe for sedation and may suppress milk supply.
Ryna liquid	Chlorpheniramine, Pseudoephedrine	Probably safe; observe for sedation and may suppress milk supply.
Ryna-C liquid	Chlorpheniramine, Pseudoephedrine, Codeine	Probably safe; observe for sedation and may suppress milk supply.

Trade Name	Ingredients	Comments
Rynatan tablets	Chlorpheniramine, Phenylephrine	Probably safe; observe for sedation.
Rynatuss tablets	Chlorpheniramine, Phenylephrine, Carbetapentane, Ephedrine	Unsafe
Singlet for adults tablets	Acetaminophen, Chlorpheniramine, Pseudoephedrine	Probably safe; observe for sedation and may suppress milk supply.
Sinutab non-drying liquid caps	Guaifenesin, Pseudoephedrine	Probably safe but may suppress milk supply.
Sinutab sinus allergy, maximum strength tablets	Acetaminophen, Chlorpheniramine, Pseudoephedrine	Probably safe; observe for sedation and may suppress milk supply.
Sinutab sinus without drowsiness maximum strength tablets	Acetaminophen, Pseudoephedrine	Probably safe but may suppress milk supply.
Sinutab sinus without drowsiness regular strength tablets	Acetaminophen, Pseudoephedrine	Probably safe but may suppress milk supply.
SINUtuss DM tablets	Guaifenesin, Dextromethorphan, Phenylephrine	Probably safe
SINUvent PE tablets	Guaifenesin, Phenylephrine	Probably safe
Sudafed cold & allergy maximum strength tablets	Chlorpheniramine, Pseudoephedrine	Probably safe; observe for sedation and may suppress milk supply.
Sudafed cold & sinus non-drowsy liqui-caps	Acetaminophen, Pseudoephedrine	Probably safe but may suppress milk supply.
Sudafed maximum strength sinus nighttime plus pain relief tablets	Acetaminophen, Diphenhydramine, Pseudoephedrine	Probably safe; observe for sedation and may suppress milk supply.

Trade Name	Ingredients	Comments
Sudafed multi-symptom cold & cough liquid caps	Acetaminophen, Guaifenesin, Pseudoephedrine, Dextromethorphan	Probably safe but may suppress milk supply.
Sudafed non-drowsy non-drying sinus liquid caps	Guaifenesin, Pseudoephedrine	Probably safe but may suppress milk supply.
Sudafed non-drowsy severe cold formula maximum strength tablets	Acetaminophen, Pseudoephedrine, Dextromethorphan	Probably safe but may suppress milk supply.
Sudafed sinus headache non-drowsy tablets	Acetaminophen, Pseudoephedrine	Probably safe but may suppress milk supply.
Sudafed sinus nighttime maximum strength tablets	Triprolidine, Pseudoephedrine	Probably safe; observe for sedation and may suppress milk supply.
Tanafed suspension	Chlorpheniramine, Pseudoephedrine	Probably safe; observe for sedation and may suppress milk supply.
Tavist allergy/ sinus/headache tablets	Acetaminophen, Clemastine, Pseudoephedrine	Unsafe
Tavist sinus maximum strength tablets	Acetaminophen, Pseudoephedrine	Probably safe but may suppress milk supply.
TheraFlu cold & cough nightTime powder	Acetaminophen, Chlorpheniramine, Pseudoephedrine, Dextromethorphan	Probably safe; observe for sedation and may suppress milk supply.
TheraFlu flu & cold medicine for sore throat, maximum strength powder	Acetaminophen, Chlorpheniramine, Pseudoephedrine	Probably safe; observe for sedation and may suppress milk supply.
TheraFlu flu & cold medicine original	Acetaminophen, Chlorpheniramine, Pseudoephedrine	Probably safe; observe for sedation and may suppress milk supply.

Trade Name	Ingredients	Comments
TheraFlu flu & cough nightTime maximum strength powder	Acetaminophen, Chlorpheniramine, Pseudoephedrine, Dextromethorphan	Probably safe; observe for sedation and may suppress milk supply.
TheraFlu flu & sore throat night time, maximum strength powder	Acetaminophen, Chlorpheniramine, Pseudoephedrine	Probably safe; observe for sedation and may suppress milk supply.
TheraFlu flu & sore throat, maximum strength powder	Acetaminophen, Chlorpheniramine, Pseudoephedrine	Probably safe; observe for sedation and may suppress milk supply.
TheraFlu flu, cold & cough and sore throat maximum strength powder	Acetaminophen, Chlorpheniramine, Pseudoephedrine, Dextromethorphan	Probably safe; observe for sedation and may suppress milk supply.
TheraFlu flu, cold & cough nightTime maximum strength powder	Acetaminophen, Chlorpheniramine, Pseudoephedrine, Dextromethorphan	Probably safe; observe for sedation and may suppress milk supply.
TheraFlu flu, cold & cough powder	Acetaminophen, Chlorpheniramine, Pseudoephedrine, Dextromethorphan	Probably safe; observe for sedation and may suppress milk supply.
TheraFlu maximum strength flu & congestion non-drowsy powder	Acetaminophen, Guaifenesin, Pseudoephedrine, Dextromethorphan	Probably safe but may suppress milk supply.
TheraFlu maximum strength flu, cold & cough powder	Acetaminophen, Guaifenesin, Pseudoephedrine, Dextromethorphan	Probably safe but may suppress milk supply.
TheraFlu maximum strength nightTime formula flu, cold & cough medicine	Acetaminophen, Chlorpheniramine, Pseudoephedrine, Dextromethorphan	Probably safe; observe for sedation and may suppress milk supply.

Trade Name	Ingredients	Comments
TheraFlu non-drowsy flu, cold & cough maximum strength powder	Acetaminophen, Pseudoephedrine, Dextromethorphan	Probably safe but may suppress milk supply.
TheraFlu non-drowsy formula maximum strength tablets	Acetaminophen, Pseudoephedrine, Dextromethorphan	Probably safe but may suppress milk supply.
TheraFlu severe cold & congestion nightTime maximum strength powder	Acetaminophen, Chlorpheniramine, Pseudoephedrine, Dextromethorphan	Probably safe; observe for sedation and may suppress milk supply.
TheraFlu severe cold & congestion non-drowsy maximum strength powder	Acetaminophen, Pseudoephedrine, Dextromethorphan	Probably safe but may suppress milk supply.
Triaminicin cold, allergy, sinus medicine tablets	Acetaminophen, Chlorpheniramine, Pseudoephedrine	Probably safe; observe for sedation and may suppress milk supply.
Triotann pediatric suspension	Chlorpheniramine, Pyrilamine, Phenylephrine	Probably safe; observe for sedation.
Tussend syrup	Chlorpheniramine, Pseudoephedrine, Hydrocodone	Probably safe; observe for sedation and may suppress milk supply.
Tussend tablets	Chlorpheniramine, Pseudoephedrine, Hydrocodone	Probably safe; observe for sedation and may suppress milk supply.
Tussi-12 tablets	Carbetapentane, Chlorpheniramine	Probably safe; observe for sedation.
Tussionex pennkinetic suspension	Chlorpheniramine, Hydrocodone	Probably safe; observe for sedation.
Tussi-Organidin-DM NR liquid	Guaifenesin, Dextromethorphan	Probably safe

Trade Name	Ingredients	Comments
Tylenol allergy sinus nightTime, maximum strength tablets	Acetaminophen, Diphenhydramine, Pseudoephedrine	Probably safe; observe for sedation and may suppress milk supply.
Tylenol allergy sinus, maximum strength tablets, gelcaps and geltabs	Acetaminophen, Chlorpheniramine, Pseudoephedrine	Probably safe; observe for sedation and may suppress milk supply.
Tylenol cold complete formula tablets	Acetaminophen, Chlorpheniramine, Pseudoephedrine, Dextromethorphan	Probably safe; observe for sedation and may suppress milk supply.
Tylenol cold non-drowsy formula gel-caps and tablets	Acetaminophen, Pseudoephedrine, Dextromethorphan	Probably safe but may suppress milk supply.
Tylenol flu maximum strength non-drowsy gelcaps	Acetaminophen, Pseudoephedrine, Dextromethorphan	Probably safe but may suppress milk supply.
Tylenol flu nightTime maximum strength liquid	Acetaminophen, Doxylamine, Pseudoephedrine, Dextromethorphan	Probably safe; observe for sedation and may suppress milk supply.
Tylenol flu nightTime, maximum strength gelcaps	Acetaminophen, Diphenhydramine, Pseudoephedrine	Probably safe; observe for sedation and may suppress milk supply.
Tylenol flu, maximum strength gelcaps	Acetaminophen, Diphenhydramine, Pseudoephedrine	Probably safe; observe for sedation and may suppress milk supply.
Tylenol multi-symptom cold severe congestion tablets	Acetaminophen, Guaifenesin, Pseudoephedrine, Dextromethorphan	Probably safe but may suppress milk supply.
Tylenol PM extra strength tablets, gelcaps and geltabs	Acetaminophen, Diphenhydramine	Probably safe; observe for sedation.
Tylenol severe allergy tablets	Acetaminophen, Diphenhydramine	Probably safe; observe for sedation.

Trade Name	Ingredients	Comments
Tylenol sinus nightTime, maximum strength tablets	Acetaminophen, Doxylamine, Pseudoephedrine	Probably safe; observe for sedation and may suppress milk supply.
Tylenol sinus non-drowsy maximum strength geltabs, tablets and gelcaps	Acetaminophen, Pseudoephedrine	Probably safe but may suppress milk supply.
Tylenol sinus severe congestion tablets	Guaifenesin, Phenylephrine	Probably safe
Vicks 44D cough & head congestion relief liquid	Pseudoephedrine, Dextromethorphan	Probably safe but may suppress milk supply.
Vicks 44E cough & chest congestion relief	Guaifenesin, Dextromethorphan	Probably safe
Vicks 44M cough , cold & flu relief liquid	Acetaminophen, Chlorpheniramine, Pseudoephedrine, Dextromethorphan	Probably safe; observe for sedation and may suppress milk supply.
Vicks DayQuil LiquiCaps multi-symptom cold/flu relief capsules	Acetaminophen, Pseudoephedrine, Dextromethorphan	Probably safe but may suppress milk supply.
Vicks DayQuil multi-symptom cold/flu relief liquid	Acetaminophen, Pseudoephedrine, Dextromethorphan	Probably safe but may suppress milk supply.
Vicks NyQuil cough syrup	Doxylamine, Dextromethorphan	Probably safe; observe for sedation.
Vicks NyQuil multi-symptom cold & flu relief LiquiCaps capsules	Acetaminophen, Doxylamine, Pseudoephedrine, Dextromethorphan	Probably safe; observe for sedation and may suppress milk supply.
Vicks NyQuil multi-symptom cold/flu relief liquid	Acetaminophen, Doxylamine, Pseudoephedrine, Dextromethorphan	Probably safe; observe for sedation and may suppress milk supply.
Vicodin Tuss syrup	Guaifenesin, Hydrocodone	Probably safe; observe for sedation.

Trade Name	Ingredients	Comments
Z-Cof DM syrup	Guaifenesin, Pseudoephedrine, Dextromethorphan	Probably safe but may suppress milk supply.
Z-Cof HC syrup	Chlorpheniramine, Phenylephrine, Hydrocodone	Probably safe; observe for sedation.
Z-Cof LA tablets	Guaifenesin, Dextromethorphan	Probably safe
Zephrex/ Zephrex LA tablets	Guaifenesin, Pseudoephedrine	Probably safe but may suppress milk supply.
Zyrtec-D 12 hour tablets	Cetirizine, Pseudoephedrine	Probably safe but may suppress milk supply.

Index

A Medication Guide for Breastfeeding Moms

A Medication Guide for Breastfeeding Moms

——————— *q* ———————

——————— *r* ———————

——————— *s* ———————

<u>Ordering information:</u>

Pharmasoft Publishing
1712 N. Forest street
Amarillo, TX, 79106-7017
USA

Hours: 8:00 AM - 5:00 PM CST

Telephone: 806-376-9900
                 800-378-1317

Fax: 806-376-9901

http://www.iBreastfeeding.com